High-Risk Sexual Behavior
Interventions with Vulnerable Populations

Evvie Becker
Elizabeth Rankin
University of Connecticut
Storrs, Connecticut

and

Annette U. Rickel
Georgetown University Medical Center
Washington, D.C.

Plenum Press • New York and London

Library of Congress Cataloging-in-Publication Data

On file

ISBN 0-306-45857-8 (Hardbound)
ISBN 0-306-45858-6 (Paperback)

© 1998 Plenum Press, New York
A Division of Plenum Publishing Corporation
233 Spring Street, New York, N.Y. 10013

http://www.plenum.com

10 9 8 7 6 5 4 3 2 1

Printed in the United States of America

Preface

In this volume, we describe how sexual behavior puts individuals at risk for a myriad of negative consequences, from sexually transmitted diseases, such as AIDS, to unwanted pregnancy. The consequences of these adverse outcomes for society as a whole are enormous, including the fiscal burden of health care costs, as well as the vicious cycle put in motion by teen pregnancy, lack of education, poverty, and the intergenerational transmission of this downward spiral. Specific interventions are described in each chapter, with attention to the needs of especially vulnerable populations.

In Chapter 1, the relationship between high-risk sexual behavior and its potential negative consequences is described. Specifically, various sexually transmitted diseases (STDs) are discussed, including HIV infection and AIDS, as well as less life-threatening but still dangerous STDs such as chlamydia, gonorrhea, and genital herpes. Teen pregnancy is examined in light of the cycle created by lack of opportunity, lack of education, and poverty. Consequences of unwanted pregnancy beyond the teen years are also noted, including the risks of child maltreatment for unwanted children.

In the second chapter, we describe some of the mediators and moderators of high-risk sexual behavior, including psychological factors, use of alcohol and other drugs, risk awareness, poverty, and a history of childhood maltreatment.

Models of prevention are discussed in Chapter 3, including general theoretical models of how humans change behavior, as well as specific models for changing high-risk sexual behavior. Tests of these models, along with specific prevention programs, are described.

Chapter 4 reviews the literature on ethnicity and social class considerations related to high-risk sexual behavior. Guidelines are suggested based on current research findings related to ethnic differences and socioeconomic factors. Alcohol and other drug use is also discussed in this context.

In Chapter 5, women's unique risks are discussed. Partner intimidation and/or violence, alcohol and other drug use, rape, history of abuse in childhood, psychological consequences of abortion, risk from partner's injected drug use, and transmission of HIV from mother to child are among the issues addressed.

Chapter 6 describes guidelines for intervention with gay men, outlining findings of research and prevention efforts with the gay community, as well as intervention and treatment of gay men with AIDS and their partners. Issues of grief and loss in the gay community are also addressed.

In writing this volume, we envisioned a world where prevention of sexual risk is the norm, and individuals make choices that enhance their lives and the lives of those with whom they are intimate. Like B.F. Skinner, we imagine a world where all individuals "are adequately clothed, fed, cared for, respected, able to make important choices, able to grow, able to learn, and able to love" (Biglan, 1993, p. 4). We are committed to finding ways to create such a world.

This work is dedicated to that vision.

Evvie Becker
Elizabeth Rankin
Annette Rickel

Acknowledgments

We would like to give special thanks to our research assistants, Jennifer Ganter and Manuel Morales, for their excellent support. We would also like to express our appreciation to the Department of Psychology at the University of Connecticut for providing us with the resources and support to complete this work. Finally, we are especially grateful to our series editor, Tom Gullotta, for his thorough reading of the manuscript and his perceptive comments, and to Mariclaire Cloutier of Plenum Press, for her editorial expertise in completing this project.

Contents

High-Risk Sexual Behavior
Interventions with Vulnerable Populations

1

What's at Stake
Consequences of Risky Sexual Behavior

What would the world look like if everyone practiced prevention in their sexual encounters? What if there were no AIDS, no syphilis, no gonorrhea? What if no one had to die of any of these diseases? What would a society be like with no unplanned or unwanted children, if mothers gave birth only when they themselves were fully developed, fully functioning adults? What if no infants were born infected with STDs? Although such goals may seem nearly impossible, this is the ideal to which this volume is dedicated: An end to the worldwide suffering caused by disease and death from STDs and a halt to the intergenerational cycles of poverty and deprivation associated with teen pregnancy. Abundant resources could be made available to support children and families in positive ways when there is no longer a need for the tertiary interventions currently required, such as medical treatment, foster care, protective services, welfare services, and a multitude of other costly remedies. This is the goal of the work described in this volume.

Although prevention of high-risk sexual behavior is a relatively new field of study, a great deal has been learned in the past two decades. In this volume, we have attempted to outline the state-of-the-art approaches that have the most probability of reducing high-risk behavior. This first chapter explains why sexual behavior puts individuals at risk for so many problems, including STDs such as AIDS, and unwanted pregnancy. The ramifications of these adverse outcomes for society are

1

discussed, including the financial burden of health care, as well as the relationships among lack of opportunity, teen pregnancy, child maltreatment, and the intergenerational transmission of these negative consequences.

Specific STDs are described, including human immunodeficiency virus (HIV) (which causes AIDS) and less life-threatening but still dangerous STDs such as chlamydia, gonorrhea, and genital herpes. Teen pregnancy is discussed within the framework of lack of opportunity, early pregnancy, lack of education, poverty, child maltreatment, substance abuse, and the intergenerational repetition of this pattern. Consequences of unwanted pregnancy throughout a woman's life are discussed, including the risks of child maltreatment for unwanted children and the psychological hazards of abortion versus those of single parenthood. The chapter concludes with an overview of the rest of the volume.

FACTORS AFFECTING PREVENTION

The spread of HIV and other STDs, as well as increasing rates of unplanned and unwanted pregnancy, results from a variety of factors. The widespread use of drugs coexisting with conditions of poverty has led to particularly high rates of transmission of all STDs, both through injection drug use and through sexual practices associated with drug use, such as the exchange of sex for drugs or money. This is particularly true for ethnic minority populations, especially African-American and Hispanic[1] communities, because of the overrepresentation of these minority groups in poverty areas (Rice, Roberts, Handsfield, & Holmes, 1991; Sabogal, Perez-Stable, Otero-Sabogal, & Hiatt, 1995; Seidman, Mosher, & Aral, 1992). In addition, adolescents and young adults engage in high rates of unprotected sexual activity with multiple partners, and many experiment with drugs, making this age group among the most vulnerable to the negative outcomes of high-risk

---

[1] We are aware of the difference in preference between the terms Hispanic and Latino among individuals of Spanish descent and among residents of various areas of the United States. We have chosen the term Hispanic because of its more inclusive meaning. However, for the purposes of the information in this volume, the two terms are interchangeable.

sexual behavior (Graham, 1994; Koniak-Griffin & Brecht, 1995; Rodgers & Rowe, 1993).

LINKING OUTCOMES OF HIGH-RISK SEX

Often, the consequences of high-risk sexual behavior have been studied independently of one another. Thus, we have scientific journals focused on AIDS or on family planning, and, too often, the interaction among researchers working on these outcomes may be minimal or nonexistent. In this monograph, we focus on high-risk sexual behavior and attempt to bridge the gap between these outcomes.

In fact, from the perspective of some populations, the gap between the various outcomes (STDs, pregnancy) may not be that large, suggesting that researchers may have created an artificial gulf between them. In a study of low-income, inner-city women in Chicago, Kalichman, Hunter, and Kelly (1992) found that study participants perceived AIDS as less worrisome than child care, crime, and employment, and about equal in concern to housing, transportation, health care, and drug abuse.

In their replication of the earlier work, Kalichman, Adair, Somlai, and Weir (1995) included inner-city men in their study, and recruited the 194 subjects from a clinic for the treatment of STDs. Most were ethnic minorities. The study found that for these men, AIDS was a primary concern; however, they were equally concerned about discrimination, crime, drug abuse, and teen pregnancy. For women in the sample, the same four problems (discrimination, crime, drug abuse, and teen pregnancy) were of greatest concern to them; however, unlike the men, they did not rank AIDS in this first tier of problems. Instead, women rated AIDS with problems they viewed as less threatening, including alcoholism and child care.

Kalichman and colleagues (1995) note that the ranking of teen pregnancy as a major concern by both men and women offers some potential for effective intervention, given that increased condom use could prevent the majority of incidences of either HIV-infection or pregnancy, as well as a myriad of STDs (although it is important to recognize that condoms are not always effective). Thus, researchers in the field of AIDS prevention are stressing the need for addressing the multiple consequences of high-risk sexual behavior in prevention campaigns.

PREVENTING PREGNANCY AND DISEASE

For youth engaging in sexual activity, birth control may be used inadequately or intermittently, if at all (Rickel, 1989). U.S. teen pregnancy rates are far higher than those of other industrialized countries, despite similar rates of sexual activity among youth (Alan Guttmacher Institute, 1986). Gonorrhea rates among U.S. adolescents more than tripled between 1958 and 1988 (Adler, 1994), STDs have reached epidemic proportions among U.S. teens, and HIV infection is increasing at alarming rates among youth (Hein, 1992).

Preventive measures include condoms, diaphragms, and other mechanical devices, as well as gels, foams, and oral contraceptives. Whereas latex condoms are the best available protection against STDs, including HIV infection, they are not necessarily the best means for preventing pregnancy, because the failure rate is greater for condoms than it is for oral contraceptives (Segest, 1994). However, studies reveal that the issue of failure rates is a complex one, and that correct use and compliance are both key factors in the success of all contraceptive measures (Rickel, 1989).

Controlled laboratory studies with latex condoms have demonstrated leakage rates in several brands of condoms. In one study, leakage rates ranged from 0.9 percent to 25.7 percent for most brands, and the shelf life of the condom did not seem to make a difference (Voeller, Nelson & Day, 1994). However, for one brand of condoms, leakage was detected in every specimen (100 percent).

In another study, latex condoms were tested with 262 U.S. couples using 4589 latex condoms from 20 lots differing in age, storage history, and laboratory testing results (Steiner, Foldesy, Cole, & Carter, 1992). Breakage rates in this study ranged from 3.5 percent for a new condom lot to 18.6 percent for condoms from an 81-month-old lot. Although laboratory testing results were found to be highly accurate in predicting condom breakage, by far the best predictor of breakage in this study was the age of the condom lot. The latter finding was an unexpected result in this study.

Yet another factor affecting condom failure rates is the use of oil-based lubricants, which have been shown to increase breakage in both new condoms and older shelf-life condoms (Steiner, Piedrahita, Glover, Joanis, Spruyt, & Foldesy, 1994). Furthermore, water-based lubricants were not only found to have no impact on new condom breakage, they also actually decreased the breakage rate of aged condoms, compared to using no lubricant. Thus, prevention programs generally stress the use of water-based lubricants only.

In addition to problems of leaking, breaking, and improper or inconsistent use, latex condoms have raised concerns because of emerging allergic responses to latex in some susceptible individuals (Stratton & Alexander, 1993). Effective condoms made of other materials are being developed. In addition, spermicides with nonoxynol-9 (N-9) as an active ingredient have been found to prevent the spread of STDs, particularly gonorrhea and chlamydia. In vitro studies had indicated that N-9 was capable of destroying HIV, and clinical trials with high-risk populations have been underway throughout the 1990s to test its efficacy for prevention of HIV infection, particularly in women (Alexander, 1996; Martin et al., 1997; Weir, Roddy, Zekeng, & Feldblum, 1995). Of concern was the possibility of vaginal irritation and ulceration resulting from the spermicide, which could make women more susceptible to HIV infection; however, controlled studies of female sex workers showed no evidence of a relationship between N-9 use and vaginal irritation or ulceration (Martin et al., 1997; Weir et al., 1995). Then, in the spring of 1997, research findings were announced that showed N-9 failed to protect against HIV-1, the most common form of the AIDS-causing virus, and the one most frequently found in the United States (Rowe, 1997).

Despite considerations regarding condom effectiveness, researchers in this field continue to point out that numerous studies have demonstrated that latex condoms used correctly and consistently are highly effective in preventing STDs, including HIV infection (Roper, Peterson, & Curran, 1993). Concerned about the mixed messages being given about condom efficacy, these authors suggest that consistent education about and promotion of condom use will prevent a great deal of human suffering. Other researchers have noted in laboratory-controlled studies that condom effectiveness at its worst is still better than not using a condom at all, by several orders of magnitude (Carey et al., 1992).

Nevertheless, the fact remains that the most effective pregnancy-prevention measures are hormonal interventions, such as oral contraceptives (i.e., birth-control pills), followed by intrauterine devices (IUDs). However, these highly effective means of preventing pregnancy also may depend upon proper and consistent use, as well as appropriate medical care and follow-up. For example, although the failure rate of oral contraceptives has been reported to be as low as 0.1 percent, this rate has been found to vary by age, race, and marital status (Hillard, 1992). Among single, black teens, the failure rate may be as high as 18 percent. Overall failure rates are believed to be about 6.2 percent in the first year of use. As Hillard points out, this can translate to a long-term failure rate of 25 to 50 percent for pregnancy in a 10-year period for individuals. The problem of compliance is the primary factor in these failures, with teens estimated to typically miss about three pills a month, and another 20 to 30 percent of users missing one pill a month.

Interventions that provide proper education regarding use and follow-up care may improve the effectiveness of these measures. One large-scale study in India provided intensive training to health care workers in counselling and motivational skills enhancement for managing patient use of contraceptives (Indian Council of Medical Research Task Force on IUD and Hormonal Contraceptives, 1994). The study followed the use of intrauterine devices in 4808 women and oral contraceptives (birth-control pills) with 1961 women for a two-year period. Results indicated that with these training programs for health care workers in place, the cumulative failure rate for the IUD after two years varied from 0.3 percent for one brand of IUD used to 0.7 percent for the second IUD brand used. Likewise, the failure rate for oral contraceptives was very low after two years, at 0.2 percent. However, the high rate of attrition for the study (20 percent for IUD and 31 percent for birth-control pills), despite intensive efforts aimed at follow-up, makes these low rates of effectiveness considerably less impressive. This problem of follow-up in India mirrors the issues found with high-risk groups in the United States, particularly those living in poverty, minority populations, and adolescents.

Another hormonal intervention, known as emergency hormonal contraception (EHC), or the so-called "morning-after" pill, is widely used in European countries. One study in London of 150 women receiving EHC (Evans, Holmes, Browning, & Forster, 1996) found that 62 percent of these women reported condom failure, 5 percent reported oral contraceptive failure, and 32 percent had used no contraception during the last intercourse (two of these women requested EHC after sexual assault). The authors noted that despite the high rate of condom failure, most of these women continued to prefer the use of condoms. They also noted that 53 percent of the women did not return to the clinic for follow-up or for contraceptive advice, suggesting that these issues must be thoroughly addressed in the initial treatment session.

In recent years, the implant known as Norplant has been introduced as yet another hormonal method of contraception. A subdermal implant (i.e., beneath the skin), Norplant is highly effective in preventing pregnancy and eliminates problems of compliance, although follow-up may still be an issue. One study of adolescents indicated a high level of interest in the use of Norplant (Dabrow, Merrick, & Conlon, 1995). Responses from 28 teen mothers and 79 teens who had never been pregnant indicated both groups had a high interest in Norplant as a means of contraception: 73 percent of the nonparenting teens and 89 percent of the adolescent mothers believed Norplant would be a better choice than oral contraceptives; 87 percent of teens without children and 81 percent of the teen moms reported they specifically liked the idea of not having to take a pill each day and the effectiveness of Norplant in pregnancy prevention.

Of course, contraceptive methods such as the IUD and hormonal interventions provide no protection from STDs. In fact, there is even some evidence that the use of hormones as oral contraceptives may increase the risk of HIV transmission because of their effect on the pathogens themselves (e.g., some bacteria have receptors for hormones; Alexander, 1996).

The fact that the research community has not always addressed these issues together is, in part, due to this basic problem of prevention strategies. If females are the primary target for prevention, then interventions are more likely to succeed when teens are encouraged to use measures they can fully control, such as taking a pill each evening at bedtime or obtaining a hormonal implant. Encouraging females to demand that male youth use condoms raises a number of issues, including insufficient assertiveness on the part of the female teen, fears she may be seen as promiscuous, and sexual self-esteem concerns; coercion or violence on the part of the male may also be a major factor in some relationships (Biglan, Noell, Ochs, Smolkowski, & Metzler, 1995; Eby, Campbell, Sullivan, & Davidson, 1995; Flores-Ortiz, 1994; van der Straten, King, Grinstead, Serufilira & Allen, 1995; Zeanah & Schwarz, 1996).

SEXUALLY TRANSMITTED DISEASES

Below are brief descriptions of the most common sexually transmitted diseases, their symptoms, treatment, and potentially damaging consequences.

Bacterial Infections

Chlamydia

In the United States, chlamydia trachomatis is the most common sexually transmitted infection (Ferreira, 1996). Although rates have been shown to be declining among college students (Cleavenger, Juckett, & Hobbs, 1996), the risk of infection remains high for adolescents, both in the United States and elsewhere (Herrmann & Egger, 1995; Oh et al., 1996). After exposure to the chlamydia bacterial organism through sexual contact (oral, anal, or vaginal), symptoms usually develop in one to three weeks; however, many of those infected experience no symptoms at all. Cleavenger and colleagues (1996) found 75.2 percent of female patients testing positive for chlamydia during a routine examination were asymptomatic; 48.8 percent of university health service patients testing positive had no symptoms. Men presenting to the health service were far more likely to have symptoms, including penile discharge, burning on urination, and/or testicular pain. When present, women's symptoms may include increased vaginal discharge, vaginal bleeding between menstrual periods, painful urination, and/or abdominal pain. Antibiotics are effective in treating chlamydia; however, it is imperative that all sexual partners receive the treatment; otherwise, the risk of reinfection is very high. The primary risk of chlamydia is *permanent infertility for both men and women.*

Trichomoniasis

Symptoms of trichomonas vaginalis, another relatively common STD, appear anywhere from five to 30 days after sexual contact. Men often have no symptoms, although a small amount of urethral discharge may be present that can easily go unnoticed (Krieger, 1995). For women, trichomoniasis is one of the most common causes of vaginitis (White, Griffith, Vetrosky, & Dixon, 1996). Women may have an odorous yellow vaginal discharge, pain with urination, vaginal irritation, or may experience painful intercourse. Treatment again must be for both partners with oral medication, if reinfection is to be avoided. Although trichomoniasis is easily treated with antibiotics, its presence has been associated with susceptibility to HIV infection, risk for delivery of low-birthweight and preterm infants, and abnormal Papanicolaou (Pap) smear screens for cervical cancer (the latter in homeless women), increasing the concern for prevention and early treatment of this relatively widespread infection (Johnstone, Tornabene, & Marcinak, 1993; Krieger, Verdon, Siegel, Critchlow, & Holmes, 1992; Murphy & Jones, 1994).

Gonorrhea

Rates of gonorrheal infection appear to be declining in some areas of the country (Hamers et al., 1995); however, some rural areas appear to be experiencing alarmingly high rates of infection (Thomas, Schoenbach, Weiner, Parker, & Earp, 1996). Increased rates of infection have also been documented in a psychiatric population (Sitzman, Burch, Bartlett, & Urrutia, 1995). Symptoms of gonorrheal infection may develop from two to 21 days after contact; however, most women and some men never experience any symptoms. When they do have symptoms, men may experience penile discharge and burning urination. Women who have symptoms may experience increased vaginal discharge, burning with urination, abnormal menstrual periods, or abdominal pain. As with many other STDs, antibiotic treatment must be given to all sexual partners to prevent reinfection. Gonorrhea has serious consequences, including permanent infertility, ectopic pregnancy, arthritis, and heart problems. As with a number of other STDs, gonorrhea can be transmitted from mother to infant during childbirth.

Syphilis

Once believed to be substantially controlled, syphilis has come back in epidemic proportions in recent years. Epidemic outbreaks have been documented in urban areas across the country, primarily among inner-city populations and crack cocaine users, particularly women (Gunn et al., 1995; Hamers et al., 1995; McFarlin & Bottoms, 1995). Consequently, the United States has experienced a surge in cases of congenital syphilis since the 1980s (Table 1.1), that is, cases of infants born with the disease transmitted by their mothers (Jonna et al., 1995; Thompson et al., 1995). In the first stage of infection, syphilis symptoms appear between nine and 90 days after contact. A sore in the mouth or genital area may appear in this first stage; however, the sore does not cause any pain, so it may not be noticed. In the second stage, four to eight weeks after the appearance of the first-stage sore, the infected person may have a rash or swollen glands. Again, these symptoms could be overlooked. Treatment with antibiotics is generally very effective;

Table 1.1. Congenital Syphilis (Infants Infected at Birth): Reported Rates in Infants Younger than One Year of Age, United States, 1980–1996[a]

Year	Rates per 100,000 live births	Year	Rates per 100,000 live births
1980	3.0	1989	44.7
1981	4.4	1990	91.0
1982	4.3	1991	107.3
1983	4.3	1992	94.7
1984	6.7	1993	80.9
1985	7.0	1994	55.8
1986	9.5	1995	47.4
1987	11.6	1996	30.4
1988	16.8		

[a]Source: Division of STD Prevention. (1997, September). *Sexually transmitted disease surveillance, 1996.* Atlanta: Centers for Disease Control and Prevention, U.S. Public Health Service.

again, such treatment must be for all sex partners. Although dwarfed in recent years by AIDS, syphilis has very serious potential complications. For that reason, prior to antibiotics the consequences of infection were extreme; in recent years, strains resistant to known antibiotics have begun to appear. Without treatment, long-term effects include brain damage, heart disease, and even death. When syphilis is passed to the fetus by an infected mother, usually in the third trimester of pregnancy, it can cause severe damage and long-term disability to the child.

Viral Infections

Human Papillomatous Virus (HPV)

HPV appears as genital warts anywhere from three weeks to six months after sexual contact with an infected person. One of the most common STDs, more than 60 types of HPV have been identified; 20 of these types have been found to cause genital warts, and the other types have a potential link to cancer (Carson, 1997). The painless warts of HPV may be found in the vaginal, anal, or penile area, and they may also appear in the mouth after oral sex. There is no cure for this virus; management of symptoms is difficult, and recurrence is likely. Affected areas are treated by removal of the warts by cryosurgery (freezing), laser, surgical excision, or with topical chemicals. In women, genital warts have been associated with precancerous changes of the cervix or genitals, as well as with cervical cancer, the second most common form of cancer in women (Kenney, 1996). Men may be at increased risk of penile cancer. Mothers may transmit the disease to their newborn during childbirth, especially since genital warts are more likely to grow during pregnancy.

Herpes Simplex Virus

Between 1966 and 1984, physician–patient consults for genital herpes increased 15-fold (Davies, 1990). Symptoms of genital herpes simplex usually occur within two to 21 days after sexual contact. Sores appear in the vaginal area, in the anal area, or on the penis. Sometimes these sores are accompanied by swollen glands in the groin area and flulike symptoms. Treatment of symptoms is with Acyclovir capsules, which sometimes reduce symptoms. However, there is no cure for the herpes virus. Infections often will reappear throughout one's life, particularly during times of stress (Swanson, Dibble, & Chenitz, 1995). During these times, the infected person can transmit herpes ("shed" the virus) to another person. Therefore, infected persons should abstain from sexual contact until all symptoms resolve. However, asymptomatic shedding may also occur. Long-term complications, in addition to persistent recurrence, involve the risk of a mother transmitting the virus to an infant during pregnancy, childbirth, and after birth (Jones, 1996). The mother often is asymptomatic when she transmits the virus to her infant. Newborns who are not promptly diagnosed and treated are at risk of serious complications, which can even lead to death.

Human Immunodeficiency Virus (HIV)

Human immunodeficiency virus (HIV) was identified as the virus causing acquired immunodeficiency syndrome (AIDS) between 1983 and 1984 by scientists working in three different laboratories in France and the United States (Kalichman, 1995). In 1986, the three discoveries were determined to be variants of the same retrovirus and were named HIV, type 1, or HIV-1. That same year, another AIDS-causing virus was discovered in West Africa, subsequently named HIV-2. Although HIV-1 and HIV-2 show differences, primarily in their molecular structure, their clinical manifestations are quite similar. HIV-1 accounts for most of the cases in the world; by 1992, 32 cases of HIV-2 had been reported in the United States, and most were West African immigrants.

In 1993, a large-scale testing of 31,533 anonymous blood specimens from high-risk populations in the United States found nearly 10 percent were positive for HIV-1; HIV-2 was found in only two heterosexual black males from a clinic for STDs (Onorato, O'Brien, Schable, Spruill, & Holmberg, 1993). Despite the low prevalence of HIV-2, the authors recommended public health surveillance testing for this virus strain, to track its invasion of the U.S. population.

By contrast, a study of 1209 female sex workers on the Ivory Coast of Africa revealed 80 percent were positive for HIV infection, and 38 percent of those infected carried both HIV-1 and HIV-2 strains of the virus (Ghys et al., 1995). The dually infected women were significantly more likely than the HIV-1 infected women to be immigrants, to have been infected with syphilis, to be age 20 or older, and to charge less for sex. The authors concluded that the greater prevalence of HIV-1 resulted primarily from earlier acquisition of that strain compared to HIV-2. Thus, the likelihood of global spread of both strains is quite high.

Symptoms of HIV infection may appear any time from two to four weeks after the virus has entered the blood stream, to several years after exposure (although the time for antibodies that produce a positive response to HIV testing to appear in the blood is usually no more than six months). The initial exposure, in some individuals, results in an acute illness which lasts one to two weeks. This reaction to primary infection manifests in flulike symptoms, including fever, sore throat, headache, lethargy, muscle weakness, light sensitivity, and eye pain. Some infected persons never experience this initial onset reaction; studies have estimated anywhere from 10 to 60 percent do not have these symptoms in the beginning stages of infection (Kalichman, 1995). However, about 70 percent of infected individuals will have enlarged lymph glands for the first few weeks of infection.

The virus itself cannot be detected through testing until at least two months after infection, when antibodies begin to appear; however, the incubation period for many people may be as long as six months, and occasionally, even two to three years. Generally, individuals who test negative but are at risk are encouraged to get a repeat testing after six months.

After the initial infection, HIV works silently in the body, replicating throughout the system, until the individual develops AIDS. Infected individuals may be symptom-free for as much as 50 to 80 percent of the time they are infected with the virus (Kalichman, 1995). Finally, after years of destruction by the virus, the immune system breaks down and can no longer protect the person from all manner of infections and diseases. Immune system cells (called "T-helper lymphocytes," or T-cells) which provide this protection are gradually destroyed by the virus. The drop in T-cell count has been found to be associated with disease progression and the onset of AIDS; however, some individuals have remained symptom-free despite extremely low T-cell counts. The diagnostic criteria for AIDS continues to be revised by the Centers for Disease Control (CDC), so that in 1993 T-cell counts below 200 cells/mm^3 in an asymptomatic individual with HIV infection became sufficient to warrant an AIDS diagnosis (U.S. Department of Health and Human Services, 1994).

At later stages of HIV infection, when T-cell counts are extremely low, individuals may experience weight loss, chronic diarrhea, persistent herpes infections of the genitals, skin rashes, and mouth, esophageal or vaginal infections. The onset of AIDS may be detected from these opportunistic infections (e.g., candidiasis infections of the throat or respiratory tract—sometimes called "thrush"), from other ailments such as pneumonia, or from cancers such as lymphomas or sarcoma, as well as from a low T-cell count.

Treatment may slow the course of HIV infection or reduce symptoms, or treatment may be directed at specific diseases or infections which arise as a result of the depleted immune system. There is no cure; death is the most common result for infected persons. However, the course of the disease is extremely variable; some individuals die within a few years of contracting the disease; others have lived for 10 years or more after becoming infected with HIV. As new treatments are instituted, infected individuals are surviving much longer than in earlier periods. Some researchers anticipate that soon HIV will become another chronic illness (e.g., like cancer or heart disease), rather than a death sentence (Beaudin & Chambre, 1996).

Mothers may infect their babies during pregnancy, childbirth, or through breast-feeding. Rates of transmission from mother to child have been estimated at 25 to 30 percent in developing countries and 14 to 25 percent in industrialized countries (John & Kreiss, 1996). Mathematical models of data suggest that 95 percent of infant infections occur later than the last two months of the pregnancy, with the risk of in utero transmission estimated at 7.7 percent, the risk of a combined in utero and at-birth transmission at 17.6 percent, and the risk of postnatal transmission at 4.9 percent. Transmission through breast-feeding is associated with a 14 percent risk, and the risk increases with longer periods of breast-feeding. Risk is greater when the mother is in the advanced stages of HIV infection and when she has been recently infected. Infants may be at greater risk when they are premature, lack cellular immunity, and when they are deficient in vitamin A. Zidovudine (AZT) treatment for the mother during pregnancy was associated with a 67.5 percent transmission risk reduction in clinical trials; this treatment has been implemented in industrialized countries but is prohibitively expensive and rarely available in undeveloped countries, where large numbers of women are infected. In Zimbabwe, for example, about 120,000 HIV-infected women are pregnant each year (Verkuyl, 1995). Furthermore, the question of whether HIV-infected mothers should be discouraged from breast-feeding in these countries, where food is scarce and formula is expensive, has become a matter of controversy and international debate.

MODES OF TRANSMISSION FOR STDs

All sexually transmitted diseases are contracted by engaging in sexual activity with an infected individual. In general, contact which places individuals at risk involves genital, anal, or oral sex between homosexual or heterosexual couples whereby the infectious organism is able to enter the tissues of the uninfected individual. In addition, in most of these STDs, mothers may transmit the disease to their unborn offspring.

In recent years, other significant aspects of these modes of transmission have begun to be recognized. For example, the presence of an STD has been increasingly documented as a marker for child sexual abuse (Derksen, 1992). That is, an STD in a young child is considered strong physical evidence supportive of sexual abuse charges in a forensic situation. Male violence against women has also recently been identified as an important factor that must be addressed in the prevention of STD transmission in women (Eby et al., 1995). When women are intimidated, coerced, or forced into sexual activity, they are unlikely to be able to attempt to introduce the use of measures protective against disease or pregnancy.

In the case of HIV infection, all of the above modalities are relevant. Although transmission through woman-to-woman sexual contact is extremely rare (Lemp et al., 1995), concern has grown for the small but significant numbers of HIV infection among women who have sex with women (White, 1997), suggesting clinicians need to be mindful of the risk factors for this group. In addition to mother-to-infant and sexual transmission, HIV may also be contracted through needle sharing with an infected individual, generally during injection drug use. Blood transfusions have also been a mode of transmission, particularly before adequate screening measures were developed.

HIV infections are linked to other STDs: a history of STDs is a strong predictor of HIV infection, over and above other predictors (Kalichman, 1995). This is not only because of the likelihood that such individuals are engaging in high rates of risky sexual behavior, but also because some STDs make HIV infection more likely. For example, genital herpes, chlamydia, and gonorrhea all cause ulcerated skin lesions which facilitate transmission of HIV, in both directions. That is, ulcerations may become entry points for the introduction of HIV, or they may be points on the HIV-infected individual where HIV cells exist in large numbers (because of the presence of immune cells fighting the co-occurring STD), ready to be transported into another person's system. Where other STDs are present, the risk of HIV infection has been shown to increase three to five times, and this is especially true for women, particularly for female drug users (Belongia et al., 1997; Gourevitch et al., 1996; Kalichman, 1995).

Most STDs have very serious consequences, ranging from infertility and transmission to newborns to systemic problems such as arthritis, heart disease, brain damage, and cancer. In some cases, death is the result. Obviously, preventing STDs would considerably reduce human suffering, health care costs, lost productivity, and loss of life.

TEEN PREGNANCY

The incidence of adolescent sexual activity has been increasing rapidly in the United States in the past few decades. As many as 21 percent of teens between the ages of 11 and 14 report having engaged in sexual intercourse (U.S. Public Health Service, 1993). By age 18, 56 percent of women and 73 percent of men report sexual intercourse, compared to 35 percent and 55 percent, respectively, in the early 1970s (Alan Guttmacher Institute, 1994; U.S. Public Health Service, 1993). Twenty-five percent of sexually active teens acquire an STD (chlamydia and gonorrhea are more common in teens than in adults). Twelve percent of young women age 15 to 19 and 21 percent of those who have had sexual intercourse get pregnant each year (Alan Guttmacher Institute, 1994).

The United States has the highest teen pregnancy rates in the industrialized world (Braverman & Strasburger, 1993; Wilcox, Rob-bennolt, O'Keeffe, & Pynchon, 1996). Rates have been documented in the United States to be more than twice those of England, Norway, and Canada, three times those of Denmark and Sweden, and seven times those of the Netherlands. However, rates of sexual activity among teens in these countries do not significantly differ from those of U.S. teens. Black U.S. teens have higher rates of pregnancy than white U.S. teens; however, white teens still become pregnant twice as often as British teens, and six times more often than their Dutch peers. (Alan Guttmacher Institute, 1986).

Furthermore, out-of-wedlock births have increased dramatically in the last 25 years, so that they now account for nearly 70 percent of all births to adolescents (Alan Guttmacher Institute, 1995). Between 1970 and 1993, the rate of births to nonmarried teens doubled, a trend with major policy implications (Wilcox et al., 1996).

A large-scale survey of 1087 high school students (10th to 12th grade; 53 percent female) found that 51 percent of these subjects reported they were sexually active (Hawkins, Spigner, & Murphy, 1990). Yet only 26 percent indicated they would seek pregnancy prevention information, and 24 percent reported they would seek information regarding prevention of HIV infection.

Recent studies with a college population indicate teen pregnancy rates may be increasing for this group. In one study, pregnancy before the age of 18 was reported by nearly 10 percent of college females at a large, state university in the northeastern United States in 1996, three times the rate reported by college women on the same campus five years earlier (Becker-Lausen & Gleeson, 1996). However, only one of the women in the 1996 study reported a live birth (information that was not available in the 1991 sample), compared to 22 reported abortions and seven miscarriages.

Impact of Teen Pregnancy on Education and Opportunity: Relationship to Poverty

Most studies indicate that more than four-fifths of adolescent pregnancies are unintentional, and that few unmarried teens plan their pregnancies (Rickel, 1989; Sidel, 1996). In her work on pregnancy intention, Adler (1994) distinguished between pregnancy intention and the motivation to *avoid* pregnancy, suggesting that the latter may be a better indicator of who is at risk for early pregnancy. She found, for example, that self-esteem level and educational aspiration were primary mediators of pregnancy outcome. Girls who have poor self-concepts and who do not see a possibility for improving their circumstances through academic achievement are more likely to view pregnancy as a viable option, and they have little reason to avoid it.

Girls who do become pregnant often do not complete their schooling, particularly if they have a second child soon after the first (Seitz & Apfel, 1993). However, poverty and lack of opportunity have repeatedly been shown to be significant factors leading to teen pregnancy, so that a cycle of poverty and hopelessness continues for children born into disadvantaged environments, where there also may be significant exposure to violence, as well (Desmond, 1994; Gordon, 1996; Sullivan, 1993).

The adolescent who is able to delay the birth of the second child has a better chance of breaking out of this cycle. One longitudinal study of teen mothers found that young women who had a second child soon after the first were four times more likely to be on welfare and 72 percent less likely to be economically secure at a 17-year follow-up point (Furstenberg, Brooks-Gunn, & Morgan, 1987). These findings suggest intervention programs for teen mothers should stress the goal of delaying a second pregnancy while the adolescent completes her schooling and develops vocational skills.

Relationship to Child Maltreatment

Studies have indicated child maltreatment may be both an antecedent and an outcome of adolescent pregnancy (Becker-Lausen & Rickel, 1995). For example, a history of sexual abuse was found to differentiate teen mothers who neglected or abused their children from those who did not (Zuravin & DiBlasio, 1992; Boyer & Fine, 1989). A recent study of mothers and children in a clinic setting found that the mothers' reports of their own child maltreatment, including reports not only of sexual abuse, but also of neglect and negative home environment, differentiated those who had substantiated abuse and neglect charges from those who had no protective services involvement (Prinos, 1996; Prinos, Becker-Lausen, & Rickel, 1997). Furthermore, a mother's current level of trauma symptoms also distinguished substantiated abuse or neglect cases from those mothers with no protective services involvement, as well as from mothers who had unsubstantiated investigations by protective services.

Child maltreatment may also be a factor in a teen's early sexual experimentation, which increases her vulnerability to becoming pregnant at a young age, continuing a negative cycle of intergenerational transmission of negative outcomes (Gleeson & Becker-Lausen, 1996; Rickel & Becker-Lausen, 1995).

In a college sample, young women who reported having been pregnant before age 18 were significantly more likely to endorse items reflecting lack of accurate knowledge about AIDS, including facts about transmission (Gleeson, 1996). Likewise, males who reported impregnating a girl before the age of 18 were significantly less likely to engage in safe sex discussions as college students.

Intergenerational Patterns

"The teen's first pregnancy may be the 'red flag' of the underlying problem of an upbringing replete with unmet basic needs . . . the problem, if not addressed, repeats, often with results far more disastrous than the first" (Rabin, Seltzer, & Pollack, 1991, p. 305). Teenage pregnancy occurs more frequently where multiple risk factors are present, including family factors such as substance abuse, violence, or divorce; individual factors such as low self-esteem; and sociocultural variables such as poverty and peer group influence (Shealy, 1995; Yawn & Yawn, 1993). In turn, adolescent mothers are less likely to complete high school and to find adequately paid jobs than mothers who begin childbearing in adulthood (Ruch-Ross, Jones, & Musick, 1992); the children of these mothers are more likely to fail in school, abuse alcohol or other drugs, and exhibit behavioral problems.

High-risk sexual behavior by adolescents, such as promiscuity or failure to use condoms, was shown to be intercorrelated in two studies by Biglan et al. (1990). In these two studies, the teens with the most risky behaviors were the least likely to use condoms. High-risk sexual behavior was also related to engaging in other unhealthy behaviors, such as the use of alcohol, drugs, and cigarettes. All of these problem behaviors were found to be related to the lack of parent availability or support.

Two new reports were released simultaneously in 1997 which support and extend these earlier findings (Lewin, 1997). Studies by the Commonwealth Fund and by the Alan Guttmacher Institute both found that one in four adolescent girls had been either sexually or physically abused or forced to have sex against her will by a dating partner. Those who reported these experiences were far more likely than the other girls to report depression and to engage in risky health behaviors such as failing to use contraception, becoming pregnant, smoking, drinking, drug use, and eating disorders. The Commonwealth Fund study surveyed 6748 girls and boys in grades 5 through 11: Girls were found to be more likely than boys to report abuse, and one in four girls said they had wanted to leave home at some point because of concerns about violence; girls were almost as likely as boys to engage in smoking, drinking, and drug use; girls reported depressive symptoms at a rate 50 percent greater than the boys, and one in three girls in high school said they had thought about suicide in the past two weeks.

The Guttmacher study analyzed survey data from 3128 girls in 8th, 10th, and 12th grades in Washington state in 1992 (Lewin, 1997). The findings indicated girls who reported they had been sexually abused were three times more likely than the other girls to have been pregnant, and that this link was primarily the result of greater sexual risk-taking on the part of the abused girls. Those with a sexual abuse history were more likely to report intercourse before age 15, more than one sexual partner, and failure to use contraception at last intercourse. In addition, the Guttmacher study showed that sexually abused girls were more likely to also report physical abuse, lack of parental supervision, school absence, lower grades, thoughts of dropping out and of suicide, and alcohol or drug use.

These findings are consistent with studies of youth delinquency, which indicate that higher levels of delinquency are present in teens in association with greater levels of maltreatment in their childhood (Smith & Thornberry, 1995; Widom, 1989). Furthermore, adolescents are more likely to engage in delinquency and drug use with increasing numbers of risk factors in their lives (Smith, Lizotte, Thornberry, & Krohn, 1995). The Smith et al. study of 1006 youth (7th to 8th grade) found that factors protecting at-risk teens from delinquency and drug use included parental supervision and attachment to a parent, as well as attachment to teachers, commitment to school, and educational aspirations.

Rickel and Becker (1997) have proposed models explaining the relationships among psychological variables, adolescent pregnancy, parenting styles, sociocultural and socioeconomic varibles, and positive or negative outcomes for children, suggesting that these intergenerational patterns are complex and multifaceted, requiring multidisciplinary and multilevel interventions. Studies by a number of researchers lend support to these models (Conger, Ge, Elder, Lorenz, & Simons, 1994; Forgatch & Stoolmiller, 1994; Whitbeck, Conger, & Kao, 1993; Whitbeck et al., 1992).

Some prevention researchers are advocating the application of substance abuse intervention technology to the prevention of high-risk sexual behavior among adolescents (Botvin, Schinke, & Orlandi, 1995). For example, prevention technology in the area of substance abuse has expanded to include cognitive behavioral interventions for improving an individual's ability to resist engaging in alcohol and other drug use, for decreasing or abstaining from use, and for preventing relapse. Noting that substance abuse and risky sexual behavior have similar etiologies and are likely to respond to similar strategies, the authors stress that interventions directed at social and psychological aspects of the behavior are most likely to be effective. (Primary cognitive behavioral approaches are discussed in Chapter 3.)

UNWANTED PREGNANCY

Unwanted pregnancy is a problem for adult women as well as for adolescents, and the implications of being unwanted may have serious ramifications for the developing child. Carrying an unwanted fetus has been shown to be a risk factor for the development of depression during pregnancy (Weissman & Olfson, 1995).

In one large-scale prospective study in Australia, mothers were interviewed immediately after the birth of a baby and again six months later (Najman, Morrison, Williams, Andersen, & Keeping, 1991). From this sample of 8556 Australian mothers, the authors found that mothers of unwanted infants had higher rates of anxiety and depression than those with wanted children; however, the magnitude of differences decreased at the follow-up interview. Noting a confound in the poorer mental health of some of the mothers of unplanned and unwanted children prior to their pregnancy, the authors reported that only a small number of the mothers with unwanted babies actually developed mental health problems.

Other studies have documented problems for the children who are born unwanted. For example, a longitudinal study in Prague, Czech Republic, has followed children through age 30 who were products of unwanted pregnancies, comparing them at each stage to matched control subjects who were born as the result of wanted pregnancies (Kubicka et al., 1995). In each of four data waves, unwanted subjects showed less positive psychosocial development, in general, than the matched controls demonstrated. However, by age 30, the differences were beginning to diminish.

The Kubicka et al. (1995) study also examined siblings (age 20 to 46) of the unplanned and of the accepted pregnancy subjects. Siblings of unplanned pregnancy subjects tended to show less favorable psychosocial outcomes, similar to those of their unplanned brothers and sisters, when compared to the siblings of control subjects. However, at the 30-year evaluation, only *female unplanned* pregnancy subjects showed greater emotional disturbance, compared to their accepted pregnancy controls. At this 30-year evaluation, the female siblings of the unplanned subjects did *not* show this higher level of emotional disturbance, when compared to the siblings of the accepted pregnancy controls.

Longitudinal findings such as those of Kubicka et al. (1995) further support earlier cross-cultural studies indicating that unwanted pregnancy is a factor in child abuse and neglect (Nakou, Adam, Stathacopoulou, & Agathonos, 1982; Williams, 1983; Zuravin, 1987). The earlier study by Nakou and colleagues, for example, examined factors in the cases of 50 abused and neglected Greek children. Among the 32 children who had siblings, the abused children were more often the result of unwanted or unplanned pregnancy. The abused group also had more perinatal problems and more illnesses in the first year of life.

In terms of the intergenerational transmission of abuse, researchers have concluded that about one-third of abused parents repeat the pattern by abusing their own children (Kaufman & Zigler, 1987).

Thus, most victims of childhood maltreatment do not abuse their children. However, others have suggested that problematic parenting patterns may be present as a result of maltreatment history for a greater number of these adults, who may lack adequate models of parenting behavior (Rickel & Becker, 1997). This may be so even when parents have the best intentions toward their children, and perhaps even when they have a conscious intention not to repeat behaviors of their own parents. These parents often appear in clinic settings, seeking guidance in childrearing (although that may not be the presenting problem), and they may be the most likely to benefit from interventions (Rickel, Dudley, & Berman, 1980).

Support for these assertions has been documented by Oliver (1993), who reviewed data from 60 studies (primarily from the United States and Great Britain), as well as original data on intergenerational transmission. The author concluded again that about one-third of child maltreatment victims repeat patterns of severely inadequate, neglecting, or abusive parenting with their own children. Taking it one step further, Oliver reported that, although a second one-third do *not* abuse or neglect their children, the remaining third are those who may be particularly vulnerable to becoming abusive or neglectful when they are experiencing a variety of psychosocial stressors. For this latter group, early support and intervention around parenting and other issues may be particularly critical.

UNPLANNED PREGNANCY, POVERTY, AND SINGLE PARENTHOOD

Early studies of urban poor and midwestern community populations have demonstrated high rates of unplanned pregnancies, with many negative consequences. Cummings and Cummings (1983) analyzed an urban sample of poor women aged 14 to 24 attending a family planning clinic. Among the 3568 white, 969 black and 524 Mexican-American women, most pregnancies were unplanned, and most subjects did not practice regular birth control.

Likewise, in a community sample of 1003 women aged 15 to 40 in Cedar Rapids, Iowa (Hillard, Shank, & Redman, 1982), researchers found that 44 percent of all pregnancies were unplanned, and that 56 percent of subjects had experienced one or more of these unplanned pregnancies. Unplanned pregnancies were most common among younger, poorer women and, particularly in adolescence, they frequently lead to single parenthood for mothers who are too often ill prepared to support their offspring (Kantor, Peretz, & Zander, 1984).

Many negative consequences have been found to accrue for children reared in a single-parent household. For example, they perform less well in school, are more likely to drop out, have lower levels of educational achievement, and have more problems finding work than children from two-parent homes (McLanahan & Sandefur, 1994). Young women reared in single-parent homes are more often found among teens who become pregnant and begin having children in adolescence. These negative consequences primarily result from the poverty associated with female-headed households, including the dramatic decline in income and other circumstances associated with divorce.

While abortion may circumvent these potentially negative consequences for the mother and her child, it is not without its own side effects. Responses following abortion are varied, and the variation has been associated with such factors as the woman's age and partner relationship, as well as the degree to which she and others in her life intended, planned, and wanted the pregnancy (Adler, 1992).

Some have suggested that bereavement, depression, and posttraumatic stress reactions occur for many women following abortion (Erikson, 1993; Kitamura, Shima, Sugawara, & Toda, 1993; Ney, Fung, Wickett, & Beaman-Dodd, 1994). However, this suggestion has been highly controversial, with many researchers arguing strongly for a lack of negative effects of abortion (Russo & Zierk, 1992; Wilmoth, deAlteriis, & Bussell, 1992). This controversy is discussed in greater detail in Chapter 5.

A large-scale analysis of U.S. state and federal data on abortions indicated women often chose abortion to optimize quality of marital and family life, and to decrease the risks of psychosocial and economic disadvantage for themselves and their families (Russo, Horn, & Schwartz, 1992). Thus, psychological effects of grieving for the lost child may be offset by the woman's reasons for choosing to abort.

One study of pregnant minority youth (Murry, 1995) examined factors influencing abortion decisions for 347 African-American and 108 Hispanic unmarried young women (age 15 to 21). Decision to end the pregnancy was related to ineffective use of contraceptives, disclosure of the pregnancy by the youth to her mother, communication about sex within the family, as well as to the family's income and church attendance. Hispanic women who chose abortion were younger at first intercourse and pregnancy than Hispanics who did not terminate their pregnancies; these differences did not appear among the African-American youth. For both ethnic groups, however, youth who decided against abortion were more likely to have family incomes at or below the poverty level.

DIFFERENTIAL RISKS FOR WOMEN VERSUS MEN

The AIDS epidemic has drawn attention to the critical nature of sexual risks for women; however, these risks are not new. For millennia, before antibiotics, before the availability and variety of contraceptive measures, and without access to abortion, women were essentially at the mercy of their sexuality. Women frequently died or suffered severe complications of pregnancy and childbirth, or from venereal diseases. In some cultures, this situation has not changed for today's women.

Yet despite the availability of preventive measures, women in the United States continue to be at great risk of numerous consequences of high-risk sexual behavior. Heterosexual sex is most risky for women, particularly for HIV infection, because of the uterine function as a receptacle for semen. Infected semen remain in the vagina, allowing more time for the virus to infiltrate. Receptive vaginal intercourse is second only to anal intercourse as the most risky form of sexual contact for transmission of HIV and other STDs (American College Health Association, 1990). In addition, surveys of sexual practices have revealed that more than 10 percent of U.S. women report the regular practice of anal intercourse with male partners (Voeller, 1991). Receptive anal intercourse is the most risky form of sexual behavior, because of the vulnerability of the walls of the rectum to damage by the penis, allowing the infectious organism to enter the bloodstream.

Other identified risk factors include the use of alcohol and drugs. Ericksen and Trocki (1992) surveyed 968 adult men and women in northern California regarding sexual practices and substance use. For women, STDs were associated with age, race, younger age at first intercourse, multiple sex partners, drinking behavior, and current symptoms of problems with alcohol. The women with drinking problems were four times more likely to have contracted STDs, and this factor was independent of all the other risk factors. Men also were more likely to have had STDs if they had a history of drinking problems and multiple sex partners. The direction of the relationship between substance use and high-risk sexual behavior is discussed in greater detail in later chapters.

For women, even condoms are a less than perfect protection, as can be inferred from the pregnancy rates associated with this method of birth control. In addition to their own behavior, women are placed at risk by male partners who fail to disclose other sexual contacts (e.g., bisexuality, sex with prostitutes, adultery), who do not reveal a positive HIV status, and who hide injection drug use and needle sharing. While men also are placed at risk by women's failure to disclose these factors, their risk is reduced by their anatomy (i.e., heterosexual males engage in insertive sex rather than receptive sex, where the infected semen may enter the blood through damaged tissue), as well as by sociocultural factors which affect decision-making around condom use. Some have suggested that women are 14 to 17 times more likely to contract HIV from men than men from women (Ward, 1993). Findings from one study suggesting a male-to-female transmission of 20 percent and a female-to-male transmission of only 1 percent have been the subject of considerable debate among researchers (Phillips & Johnson, 1992).

In the United States, women are among the fastest growing groups becoming infected with HIV through sexual contact or from injection drug use (Centers for Disease Control, 1993). Black and Hispanic women are especially at risk. Despite the lack of risk from woman-to-woman sexual contact, many lesbian women may also be at high risk for HIV transmission (Lemp et al., 1995). One study of 1086 lesbian and bisexual women found that 53 percent of self-defined lesbians reported sexual experiences with men since 1978, and 21 percent of lesbians reported either using injection drugs or engaging in high-risk sexual contact with gay/bisexual men or injection drug users in that time frame; for bisexual women, the percentages were 90 and 49 percent, respectively (Einhorn & Polgar, 1994).

Globally, women comprise 40 percent of adults infected with HIV (Mann, Tarantola, & Neter, 1992), although in Sub-Saharan Africa infection rates for men and women are equal, and in other parts of the world the ratios are rapidly equalizing. By the year 2000, more than 13 million women are expected to be infected with HIV and 4 million women will have died from AIDS (Ankrah, 1995). In 1985, 10 men became infected for every woman who acquired the virus; by 2000, the rate of transmission for women is expected to exceed that of men.

PREGNANCY CONSEQUENCES

Clearly, women most often bear the brunt of unplanned pregnancies, including increased rates of depression, poverty, single parenting, and abortion decisions. Wyatt and Riederle (1994) have outlined five beliefs about women's sexual behavior that they suggest are myths, and which interfere with effective prevention efforts for women. They present research findings that support the assertion that it is a myth that (1) women in general have sufficient knowledge of their sexuality to address their own needs; (2) women are able to effectively communicate about sex; (3) women are sexually active because they want to have sex; (4) sexually active women engage in sex because they enjoy it; and (5) women who know about preventive measures will use their knowledge to protect themselves against STDs and pregnancy.

Ward (1993) noted that the HIV epidemic among women in the United States is a "different disease" than HIV among men, primarily because of factors unique to the lives of poor women, the most vulnerable group. "To be poor and female in America," she writes, "is to be invisible and impotent. Long before HIV, women lost babies, had sexually transmitted diseases and needed better health and health care than they were ever likely to receive. A cure or prevention of HIV infections will not cure or prevent poverty" (p. 428).

These realities of poor women's lives today make intervention all the more difficult, for they suggest that multisystemic, multidisciplinary, multilevel approaches will be required to impact the trend toward increasingly high rates of infection and of unplanned pregnancy.

Ward (1993) concludes ironically: "The condoms manufactured and marketed for use by men have names which imply virility, power, or mythical heroes (Trojans, Ramses). The newly approved and expensive condom for females is simply called 'Reality'" (p. 428).

SUMMARY AND CONCLUSIONS

In this chapter the devastating costs to the individual and to society of high-risk sexual behavior have been outlined. STDs, including AIDS, take their toll in human suffering, health care costs, loss of productivity, illness, and death. Pregnancy that comes too soon in the mother's life and is unplanned or unwanted costs the mother and the child in economic and in psychological outcomes. Child maltreatment is both an antecedent of ill-timed pregnancy and a consequence. Society incurs costs of untimely pregnancies in terms of lost human potential and lost productivity, as well as health care and social welfare costs. Women, particularly poor and ethnic minority women (who are differentially at risk only because of their overrepresentation in poverty), are especially vulnerable to the negative outcomes associated with high-risk sexual behavior, and they are often the least able to protect themselves.

OUTLINE OF THE MONOGRAPH

In the next chapter, factors associated with engaging in high-risk sexual behavior will be explored in further detail. Chapter 2 describes what research tells us about the causes, the mediators, and the moderators of high-risk sexual behavior. Factors discussed include psychological aspects, such as low self-esteem and external locus of control; use of alcohol and other drugs; knowledge and awareness of sexual risks and prevention measures; poverty and lack of opportunity; and a history of maltreatment in childhood.

In Chapter 3, a model of stages of behavioral change is described as a foundation for understanding which type of interventions is most effective at various phases of change. Various prevention models currently in use are discussed, including Fisher's Information-Motivation-Behavioral Skills (IMB) model. This model has been tested with college students, another high-risk population discussed here. Teen pregnancy prevention efforts, as well as interventions with teen mothers that encourage school completion and delay of second pregnancy, are also outlined.

Taking into consideration current research knowledge, Chapter 4 presents guidelines for interventions with special attention to ethnic differences and socioeconomic factors as they relate to individual risk, motivation, and potential for change. Alcohol and other drug use is discussed in this context.

Special issues related to women's risks are discussed in Chapter 5, including partner intimidation and/or violence, rape, history of abuse in childhood, psychological consequences of abortion, alcohol and other drug use, risk from partner's injection drug use, and transmission of HIV to fetus.

Prevention efforts with the gay community are described in Chapter 6, as well as intervention and treatment of gay men with AIDS and their partners. Although considerable behavior change has occurred in this population, there is still a major risk of infection. Research findings are presented which highlight factors such as a history of childhood maltreatment, alcohol and other drug use, partner's use of intimidation and/or violence, especially in a sexual context, and issues of grief and loss in the gay community.

Research presented throughout the volume tends to emphasize prevention of HIV infection, because so much attention has been focused on that outcome since its discovery in the 1980s. Sex practices that prevent AIDS, however, also serve to prevent other STDs, and to a lesser extent, unplanned pregnancy. Therefore, STDs should be considered to be included as an outcome affected by most of the prevention techniques discussed herein.

The political aspects of prevention have not been addressed in this volume, as that is beyond the intention of this monograph. Practical, useful strategies and interventions are presented that hold promise for decreasing the spread of disease and the effects of untimely pregnancy. Implementation of these prevention programs will be up to the innovative and courageous individuals and groups working within their own communities, attempting to address the concerns of parents and school boards, among other interested parties.

2

Factors that Influence
Sexual Behavior
Causes, Mediators, and Moderators of
High-Risk Sexual Behavior

The tendency to engage in high-risk sexual behavior may be influenced by a number of factors. In this chapter, we will examine the effects of psychological variables, such as low self-esteem, locus of control, dissociation, and denial, on sexual practices. We will also look at the evidence for effects of alcohol and other drugs on sexual behavior. The ways in which poverty and the associated lack of opportunity impact risky behavior will be discussed, as will the effects of lack of knowledge about sex, about reproductive biology, and about their associated risks.

CHILD MALTREATMENT AND HIGH-RISK
SEXUAL BEHAVIOR

Child maltreatment is well documented as a precursor to sexual problems, including issues with sexual adjustment, sexual self-esteem, and high-risk behaviors (Browne & Finkelhor, 1986). In this section, we will discuss some of the theories and findings related to this phenomenon. We will also discuss dissociation in detail because this psychological outcome of child maltreatment (particularly sexual and

31

physical abuse) has been shown to be a key link between child abuse and adult high-risk sexual behavior.

Child abuse is a problem of huge proportions in the United States. Physical abuse and neglect account for 2000 deaths of children every year, or approximately five deaths each day (U.S. Advisory Board on Child Abuse and Neglect, 1995). As large as these numbers are, according to the U.S. Advisory Board on Child Abuse, they are probably a gross underestimation of the actual number of deaths resulting from child abuse. This group estimates that about 85 percent of deaths caused by abuse and neglect are actually attributed to unintentional causes. Twice as many children die from child abuse as die in automobile accidents. In addition, child abuse results in more than 140,000 injuries per year. Approximately 2.9 million reports of suspected abuse are made to authorities each year, concerning 1.9 million children. Nearly 1 million of these cases are substantiated.

Psychological outcomes of childhood trauma are varied and may be quite severe (Rickel & Becker, 1997). During childhood, victims of maltreatment may experience depressive symptoms such as sad affect, poor self-esteem, guilt, and helplessness. Other problems include anxiety and phobias, the inability to trust others, and social withdrawal. Problems with language development, lowered cognitive performance, and failure to thrive may be related to child maltreatment. Aggression, manifested as violence, animal abuse, and self-destructive behaviors, is also sometimes indicative of a history of child maltreatment.

In adolescence and adulthood, a history of trauma may lead to dissociation and related disorders, depression, and personality disorders (Rickel & Becker, 1997). There may also be problems with eating disorders and substance abuse. These forms of psychopathology may actually represent the use of a strategy that once proved useful in coping with the stress associated with the trauma while it was ongoing. However, the behavior, once learned, is retained, even though it may now be destructive and no longer serves its original purpose as a protective mechanism for the victim.

Dissociation

Dissociation is one such strategy that is extremely useful in coping with trauma, but in adulthood may be maladaptive. Becker-

Lausen, Sanders, and Chinsky (1995) found dissociation to be a mediator between childhood maltreatment and later revictimization. In their study, 301 college students completed the Child Abuse and Trauma (CAT) scale (Sanders & Becker-Lausen, 1995), a self-report measure of physical and sexual abuse, as well as experiences of neglect and negative home environment during childhood. Subjects were also given a measure of dissociation (Bernstein & Putnam, 1986) and one of depression (Beck, 1972), as well as measures of life outcomes, including problems with interpersonal relationships.

Becker-Lausen et al. (1995) found that dissociation, depression, and negative experiences were related to reports of child maltreatment history. Furthermore, dissociation and depression were related to different types of interpersonal difficulties. More depressed subjects tended to report social difficulties, but they showed a heightened awareness of their problems. Dissociative subjects also reported interpersonal difficulties, but they were more likely to express a lack of awareness or insight into the mechanisms underlying these problems. Depression and dissociation were related to experiencing later negative life events. Structural analyses supported the prediction that child maltreatment leads to these subsequent problems. Dissociation, for example, was related to becoming pregnant or having an abortion while in high school, academic problems such as failing a test or being placed on academic probation, or getting fired from a job.

Kluft (1990b) conceptualized dissociative individuals as "sitting ducks" for revictimization experiences. From the experience of child abuse, individuals learn to dissociate from the physical or psychological pain occurring during the abuse as it is happening. Unfortunately, this strategy becomes generalized for the child as he or she grows up. The child becomes accustomed to tuning out stimuli from the environment, even when the stimuli offer valuable information about dangers that are important to avoid. As a result, such a child or (later) adult is vulnerable to threats that other individuals recognize and negotiate to avoid being victimized.

Becker-Lausen et al. (1995) gave subjects the opportunity to rate their later experiences as either positive or negative. They found that subjects who dissociated tended to characterize their experiences in unusual ways. For example, one individual reported experiences that included serious medical problems of close relatives, yet described these experiences as positive. Kluft (1990a) described this characteristic of dissociative individuals as "dichotomous thinking," a tendency to view events as either all positive or all negative.

Dissociative identity disorder, which was called multiple personality disorder before the publication of DSM-IV (American Psychiatric Association [APA], 1994), is another extreme outcome of dissociation related to trauma (Becker-Lausen et al., 1995). This disorder is characterized by two or more different personalities which act independently of one another and which have separate identities existing within the same individual (APA, 1994).

Gleeson and Becker-Lausen (1996) found that subjects with histories of child abuse were more likely to consider the use of HIV-prevention strategies as potentially detrimental to an intimate relationship. Furthermore, subjects with elevated levels of dissociation tended to know less about AIDS risk and prevention than did others. Perhaps these individuals absorb less information about HIV prevention because the topic brings up memories of past abuse experiences and thereby activates the tendency to use dissociation as a defense.

Borderline Personality Disorder

In extreme cases, some victims of childhood abuse may develop borderline personality disorder (van der Kolk, 1996). Van der Kolk developed a hypothesis with Herman (Herman & van der Kolk, 1987) regarding the etiology of borderline personality disorder: Suffering continued abuse perpetrated by adults who are also primary caregivers leads to a reorganization of one's cognitions about oneself and other people. Van der Kolk explains: ". . . the characteristic splitting of the self and others into 'all good' or 'all bad' portions represents a developmental arrest—a continued fragmentation of the self and a fixation on earlier modes of organizing experience" (p. 201).

Borderline personality disorder is characterized as an enduring psychological disturbance marked by problems with relationships, perceptions of the self, and emotional patterns (American Psychiatric Association, 1994). Relationships are likely to be short-lived and volatile, with perceptions of the other person alternating between extremes of good and bad. Impulsive sexual behavior is characteristic, as is poorly regulated behavior in regard to finances, drug and alcohol use, and eating.

Herman and van der Kolk (1987) found that borderline personality was related to the most extreme cases of physical and sexual abuse in their clinical sample, with most of those diagnosed with borderline personality disorder having been abused before the age of 6. Thirteen percent of those subjects who were identified as having borderline personality disorder reported no history of child abuse. However, van der Kolk points out that about half of these subjects were not able to recall their childhoods very well at all, calling their self-reports into question. He found a small number of subjects diagnosed with borderline personality disorder who seemed to, in fact, have no history of abuse. He describes these subjects as having been especially shy and fearful during childhood. Based on these findings, van der Kolk conceptualizes borderline personality disorder as resulting from "having been chronically terrified during one's early development" (p. 202).

Teen Pregnancy: Risk Factors and Personality Functioning

The Detroit Teen Parent Project (Rickel, 1989) was designed to answer questions concerning the personality and situational variables that are predictive of teen pregnancy, as well as to determine how such variables are related to effective and ineffective ways of parenting for teens who have children. Subjects for the study were recruited through two high schools that served populations of pregnant or parenting adolescent girls. One of the schools allowed pregnant girls to be enrolled through the school year when they gave birth. This school provided a variety of services to girls enrolled there. These included medical services, day care, parenting instruction, and counseling. The other school allowed girls to stay through high school graduation. There were 124 subjects in all, ranging in age from 14 to 19, with a mean age of 16.1 years. The sample was ethnically mixed, with slightly more than half of the sample being African American and the remainder being white.

The study examined the teen mothers' background, levels of stress and social support, parenting skills, and personality functioning. The Rickel Modified Child Rearing Practices Report (RMCRPR) (Block, 1965; Rickel & Biasatti, 1982) was used to assess parenting style. The RMCRPR is a questionnaire that distinguishes a combination of authoritarian parenting and strictness, labeled "restrictiveness," from "nurturance," which is parenting characterized by warmth and supportiveness. Nurturance has been found to predict a number of positive outcomes, whereas restrictiveness has been related to negative outcomes for the child (Jones, Rickel, & Smith, 1980). A measure of social support networks asked the subject to identify those people in her life to whom she turned for support and the manner in which these individuals are supportive. Other measures assessed the degree of the mothers' tendencies to use positive and negative reinforcements to influence their children's behavior, their understanding of child development, and their beliefs about children and child behavior. The Minnesota Multiphasic Personality Inventory (MMPI), a standard, widely used, well-validated personality test, was used to measure personality functioning of these subjects.

Most of these girls came from families with parental divorce or separation or had parents who had not been married (Rickel, 1989); only 26 percent came from families with two parents living together. This finding may have important implications for social support, considering that families with only one parent may have fewer resources with which to support a teenage daughter who becomes pregnant.

More than 90 percent of the sample expressed a belief in God, and more than half reported going to church regularly. Many of those who endorsed the highest levels of religiosity were either Catholic or Baptist, leading the author to hypothesize that religious beliefs may have been a factor in not using birth control or in deciding to keep their babies. Seventy-seven percent of the sample were pregnant for the first time, while 18 percent were pregnant for the second time; for 2 percent the current pregnancy was their third.

While over half of the girls reported difficulties related to parenting and continuing in school at the same time, 27.2 percent reported plans to continue their education, with 6.4 percent planning to go to trade school, 19.1 percent intending to go to college, and 2.3 percent wishing to continue their education to the graduate level.

Eighty-five percent of the subjects reported that their pregnancies had been unplanned. Only about one-quarter reported being happy about their pregnancies, with 59 percent reporting fearfulness or other negative reactions to being pregnant. However, half of the subjects reported that the fathers of their children had positive reactions to their pregnancies.

Rickel (1989) used five classifications for personality outcomes on the MMPI: (1) normal, which consisted of all MMPI scales within the normal range; (2) neurotic, indicating higher scores on either depression or anxiety; (3) characterological, defined as having higher levels of rebelliousness and less acceptance of authority; (4) socially alienated, indicating higher levels of isolation and being seen by others as behaving outside accepted norms; and (5) unclassified, meaning that scale scores were elevated but not according to any one of the patterns described above.

Analyses of personality factors and their effect on parenting indicated that depression, as measured by the MMPI, was related to lower levels of parental nurturance. In addition, those subjects classified as neurotic scored lower on nurturance than did subjects falling into the other four classifications of MMPI scores, and they also tended to score lower on parental restrictiveness than subjects from the other four groups, indicating their parenting styles may be characterized by disengagement with their babies. Finally, those who were classified as socially alienated scored higher on restrictiveness.

Personality Function Related to Teen Pregnancy

In a later study, Thomas and Rickel (1995) examined MMPI scores in relation to teen pregnancy. Their study included 420 high school students, 179 of whom were either pregnant at the time of the study or already had children. The remaining subjects were not pregnant, nor were they already parents, but were control subjects from the feeder schools from which the pregnant/parenting teens originally came.

Psychopathology was much higher for the teen pregnancy and parent group, with 79 percent of these subjects scoring above the normal range on the MMPI. These subjects had elevated scores on Scale 4 (Psychopathic Deviance), Scale 5 (Masculinity/Femininity), Scale 6 (Paranoia), Scale 8 (Schizophrenia), as well as on the L and F Scales, 2 of the 3 validity Scales for the MMPI. In contrast, the control subjects tended to score low on these scales.

Teen Pregnancy and Child Maltreatment History

Although there is little existing research linking a history of child maltreatment with teen pregnancy as an outcome, there are similarities between MMPI profiles of victims of abuse and teens who have become pregnant (Rickel & Becker, 1997), suggesting that child maltreatment might be predictive of future teen pregnancy. Hunter (1991) found that adults who had experienced child abuse had high scores on Psychopathic Deviance (Scale 4), Paranoia (Scale 6), and Schizophrenia (Scale 8), as did teens who had become pregnant in Thomas and Rickel's (1995) study.

In addition, Hunter's subjects with abuse histories had scores more than two standard deviations above the mean on Psychopathic Deviance (Scale 4) and Schizophrenia (Scale 8). Hunter's subjects had scores higher than those of control group subjects on most of the other scales as well, including the K scale (the third validity scale), Hypochondriasis (Scale 1), Depression (Scale 2), Hysteria (Scale 3), Psychasthenia (Scale 7), Mania (Scale 9), and Social Introversion (Scale 0). Hunter also found that survivors of child abuse were more likely to experience poor self-esteem and problems related to sexual adjustment and relationships with others.

Based on these similarities and the study described above of factors mediating child maltreatment outcomes (Becker-Lausen et al., 1995), Becker-Lausen and Rickel (1995) proposed a model suggesting that teen pregnancy may be one potential outcome of child maltreatment.

Further evidence for this model may be found in the similarities between symptoms resulting from childhood abuse, described by Briere (1992), and the manifestations commonly associated with the MMPI scales which have been related to both child maltreatment and teen pregnancy. For example, dissociation may be related to high scores on the Schizophrenia (Scale 8) scale of the MMPI. Graham (1993) describes individuals with high Scale 8 scores as "confused, disorganized and disoriented" (p. 73), as well as possibly demonstrating "extremely poor judgment" (p. 74). He also suggests that they may have sexual issues.

Briere (1992) identifies hypervigilance as characteristic of a victim of abuse, and elevated scores on the MMPI Paranoia scale (Scale 6) may be indicative of the same symptomology. Graham (1993) describes these individuals as "angry and resentful" and "suspicious and guarded" (p. 69), which may also reflect trust issues frequently noted in abuse victims (Becker-Lausen & Mallon-Kraft, 1997; Briere, 1992). Psychopathic Deviance (Scale 4) may reflect disillusionment with the stereotypic views of family life, and by extension, with the larger society as well, because of the failure of their own families and others to meet such ideals or to protect them from harm. Graham (1993) describes the characteristics of someone who scores high on this scale as having "difficulty incorporating the values and standards of society" and being "rebellious toward authority figures" (p. 65).

Based on these similarities, Becker-Lausen and Rickel's (1995) model (Fig. 2.1) suggests that: (1) Child maltreatment results in dissociation (which may be seen as an elevated Schizophrenia [Scale 8] score on the MMPI), which, in turn, may be a mediator of pregnancy during adolescence. (2) Child maltreatment also results in higher Psychopathic Deviance (Scale 4) scores (which may be interpreted as a rejection of society's ideals and a resulting rejection of authority), which also may mediate teen pregnancy. (3) Child maltreatment causes low self-esteem, which mediates both teen pregnancy and depression. (4) Finally, child maltreatment leads to hypervigilance (which is seen as higher scores on Paranoia [Scale 6] on the MMPI), which may be associated with either teen pregnancy or depression. Ongoing research (Rankin & Becker-Lausen, 1997) is currently in progress to test some of these proposed pathways.

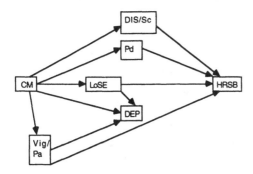

Figure 2.1. Model of child maltreatment and high-risk sexual behavior (adapted from Becker-Lausen & Rickel, 1995. Reprinted with permission). CM, child maltreatment; Pd, psychopathic scale; DEP, depression; Vig/Pa, vigilance/paranoia scale; LoSE, low self-esteem; HRSB, high-risk sexual behavior; DIS/Sc, dissociation/schizophrenia scale.

Other Psychological Factors: Low Self-Esteem

For adolescents, low self-esteem is thought to be related to high-risk sexual behavior (including early onset of sexual activity and unprotected sex), as well as substance use, accidental injuries, intentional injuries by others, and inadequate personal care, including cleanliness and dietary habits (Friedman, 1989). Emans (1983) suggests that high levels of sexual activity among adolescents results from low self-esteem and lack of cognitive development, as well as from the individual's moral development and level of maturation.

Sexual activity among adolescent girls has been found to be related to low self-esteem and lower educational goals (Adler, 1994). Earlier research by Jessor and Jessor (1975) indicated that sexually active adolescents performed worse in school than their peers and considered affection more important than their peers did. They were also more likely to have less satisfying relationships with their parents.

Davidson and Moore (1994) found evidence for relationships among risky sexual behavior, low self-esteem, and sex guilt in a population of college women. Those who reported higher levels of guilt also reported being somewhat passive in sexual decision-making. These subjects were more likely to report being uncomfortable with their sexuality and to have engaged in more risky sexual encounters than subjects who did not report feelings of guilt. More generally, subjects high in guilt reported that their feelings about their own self-worth were enhanced when someone else made decisions for them.

In a population of college men, self-esteem was found to be related to attitudes toward condom use and to an internal locus of control regarding health issues (Cole & Slocumb, 1995). The authors suggest incorporating these psychological factors into the design of more effective prevention programs for reducing risky sexual behavior.

For gay and bisexual men, low self-esteem is also related to risky sexual behavior (Paul, Stall, & Davis, 1993). One study compared gay and bisexual men who were in substance abuse treatment to a group of gay and bisexual men who were not in treatment for substance abuse. Those in the treatment group reported much higher levels of risky sexual behavior. Paul et al. propose that substance abuse contributed to this pattern of behavior through the dynamics of addiction (which serve to maintain low self-esteem), beliefs about the disinhibition of substance use, and the association of substance use with sexual activity. Passivity and a limited sense of power may also be factors in these dynamics, they suggest.

Locus of Control

Locus of control (LOC) is defined as an individual's tendency to credit the events in his or her life either to internal causes (e.g., one's own intelligence, effort, or strength, or the lack of such qualities) or to external causes (e.g., the power or actions of others, or luck) (Rotter, 1966). LOC appears to be related to individuals' beliefs about sexual choices. Dignan (1979) assessed locus of control in college students, in relation to their attitudes toward contraceptive use. He found that males tended to be more internal overall, but that female subjects who scored relatively high on internality were more likely to think of contraceptives as a means of preventing pregnancy. In another study, Dignan and Adame (1979) were able to achieve changes in locus of control toward greater internality through the implementation of a sex education program for undergraduates.

Denial

Like dissociation, denial in victims may be related to repeat victimization experiences. In a study of women from a college community, Roth, Wayland, and Woolsey (1990) found that those who had been sexually assaulted were much more likely to have psychiatric problems. Denial was related to revictimization among the women in this study.

Hooper (1989) describes denial as part of a normal process for mothers who learn that a child has been sexually abused by the mother's male partner. She describes a sequence of events that women in this situation typically experience, beginning with suspiciousness, followed by confrontation, denial, and doubt. She stresses the need for education about sexual abuse and the need to provide support for mothers caught in these situations.

Knowledge and Awareness of High-Risk Behaviors

Many adolescents in the United States receive some formal training about sex through sex education classes (Rickel, 1989). However, these efforts appear to have insufficient impact on problems like teen pregnancy. Sex education courses may prove ineffective because they fail to take students' levels of cognitive development into account, or the material may be taught in such a way that students fail to grasp the application to their own lives.

Swedish sex education programs appear to be much more effective, as evidenced by the declining rate of teenage pregnancy in that country (Rickel, 1989). In contrast to American sex education curricula, Swedish students are given information about sex, but this information is offered in a context of considerations about relationships and ethical values. Furthermore, students are encouraged to examine their own views and are aided in developing their own personal values related to sexuality and relationships.

Knowledge is also essential to the prevention of the spread of HIV, particularly for members of high-risk groups. The American Red Cross designed a program to assess levels of knowledge and to raise the awareness of African-American adolescents (Damond, Breuer, & Pharr, 1993). In this training program, efforts were made to incorporate and make use of existing cultural standards and perceptions in designing the program. Cultural considerations were also incorporated into the delivery of the program by using African Americans to conduct the training in African-American neighborhoods.

Even though the intended audience was African-American youth, other ethnicities were included because subjects were drawn from a diverse school system in Los Angeles. The sample consisted of 339 African-American, Latino, and white students ranging in age from 13 to 18 years.

Subjects completed instruments which measured both knowledge and intentions to engage in or change certain behaviors before and after the training. The knowledge questionnaire included items related to mechanisms of transmission of HIV. The questionnaire included false items for the purpose of discovering erroneous beliefs that adolescents might hold related to HIV transmission. The training consisted of one session of HIV education lasting approximately two hours.

The knowledge instrument was scored on a scale from 0 to 13. Overall, knowledge was quite high before the training, with an average score for the entire sample of 11.48, and a standard deviation of 1.47. The overall score on the intentionality measure, on a scale from 0 to 7, was 3.97, with a standard deviation of 1.76. Postintervention scores showed some improvement, with an increase in the level of knowledge to a mean of 12.11, with a standard deviation of 1.23. Intentionality was also affected by the training, with a postintervention mean of 4.63, and a standard deviation of 1.79.

There were slight differences in knowledge levels among ethnic groups. Whites had more knowledge than African Americans, who in turn demonstrated more knowledge than Latinos. This pattern was true for pre- and postintervention tests. Female subjects had slightly more knowledge than males, both before and after the training.

Differences also existed among ethnicities on the measurement of intentions. White subjects showed the highest levels of intent to engage in actions consistent with facts about AIDS transmission. Latinos had the next highest scores on this dimension of the evaluation, and African Americans had slightly lower scores. Although the scores rose from pre- to postintervention testing for all three ethnicities, the relative order of scores across ethnic groups remained the same postintervention.

The intervention produced significant changes in knowledge for several test items. For example, one item stated that AIDS had in the past been largely confined to gay and injection drug–using populations and would probably remain so in the future; fewer subjects endorsed this item postintervention. Subjects also demonstrated increased awareness that an individual's HIV status could not be determined by their appearance. Other items showing increases in knowledge after the intervention included whether HIV could be transmitted through mosquito bites or by giving blood.

Intentions were also changed by the intervention. Subjects reported greater willingness to delay having sex, sit near or administer first aid to an HIV-positive individual, give blood, use condoms, refrain from needle-sharing, and get tested for HIV.

In another study of adolescents, Davis and Harris (1982) assessed sexual knowledge of Hispanic, Native American, and white youth, ranging in age from 11 to 18 years. These 288 public school students (185 females, 103 males) were recruited from both rural (158 students) and urban (130 students) schools, so that the effects of living in each of these environments could be compared.

The questionnaire included items related to knowledge regarding sex, the resources providing this knowledge, areas of interest related to sexual matters, and questions subjects had about sex. The administration of the questionnaire represented the beginning of a course in sex education which was to be delivered to this population of students.

Across all three ethnic groups, both genders, and both urban and rural settings, subjects reported receiving most of their knowledge about sex from friends. For all nonwhite ethnic groups, school was the second most frequently cited resource (white youth ranked parents as second). For the overall sample and for female subjects, parents ranked as the third source of knowledge. However, for male subjects, movies, books and magazines, and siblings were rated higher than parents as sources of knowledge about sex. For Hispanics and African Americans, movies ranked after school and before parents. Urban subjects rated school second and parents third. For rural subjects, school and parents tied for second place, with movies running a close third.

Female subjects had higher levels of sexual knowledge than males, as well as greater interest in a larger number of sexual terms. White subjects possessed higher levels of knowledge, followed by Hispanic and Native American subjects. Davis and Harris (1982) suggest that this finding, along with the fact that white subjects reported receiving more information, might indicate that knowledge differences are related to cultural norms about the discussion of sexual matters.

Twenty-three percent of the overall sample did not know the meaning of the word condom. Other terms that were less well known included IUD, masturbation, erection, Ceasarean section, diaphragm, ejaculation, menopause, orgasm, and pornography. Fewer than half of the Native American subjects knew the terms IUD, masturbation, ejaculation, menopause, and pornography. The least well-known term for Hispanic subjects was IUD, which was unfamiliar to 47.9 percent. For white subjects, IUD was also the least familiar term, being known only by 24.5 percent. Urban students had more knowledge of sexual terms than did rural students. Likewise, older subjects possessed more knowledge than younger ones.

Davis and Harris (1982) suggest that differences across age, gender, ethnicity, and urban versus rural upbringing be considered and accommodated into the design of sex education programs. Information related to students' levels of knowledge, sources of information, and topics of interest can provide clues as to areas in which particular groups of students might be lacking in knowledge or might have received erroneous information.

Alcohol and Drug Use

The use of alcohol and other drugs is likely to lead to involvement in riskier sexual behaviors than might otherwise be considered (Kalichman et al., 1995). In addition, injection drug users and sex partners of injection drug users are at risk for contracting HIV, and users of crack face particularly great threats of becoming infected (Longshore & Anglin, 1995).

Kalichman et al. (1995) surveyed patients at a clinic that treated sexually transmitted diseases, asking about their current risky behaviors and their perception of AIDS in relation to other problems faced by their community. Alcohol use during the past month was reported by 74 percent of men and 57 percent of women; marijuana use during the past month by 49 percent of men and 31 percent of women. Cocaine use rates for men and women were 17 percent and 6 percent, respectively.

Injection drug use (IDU) was somewhat lower in this sample. IDU was reported by 6 percent of men and 2 percent of women; 9 percent of men and 7 percent of women reported having sex with someone who injected drugs. Exchanging sex for money or drugs was more common, with 32 percent of men and 13 percent of women having participated in such transactions.

Longshore and Anglin (1995) examined the validity of current beliefs that crack use by itself is an indicator of very high sexual risk. They questioned whether it is crack use per se or high-risk behaviors practiced by many of those who use crack that account for the high rates of HIV infection for this subgroup of drug users. Such risky behaviors include engaging in sexual activity in exchange for money, having sex while using alcohol or other drugs, and the use of alcohol or marijuana, in general.

Subjects for the study included adults arrested in Los Angeles. The study included more than 1700 complete interviews, with 920 subjects who were crack users and 849 who were not. There were considerably more men in the sample than women: 1151 men compared to 618 women.

The study showed that both male and female crack users had higher numbers of sexual partners than did those subjects who did not smoke crack. Crack use itself, not just the typically associated high-risk behaviors, was found to be predictive of HIV risks related to number of sexual partners, for both genders. Longshore and Anglin (1995) point out that this finding about men's risk is important, because previous studies have focused on female crack users and their high numbers of sexual partners. Demographic characteristics that are predictive of higher numbers of partners include younger age and higher income. Among male subjects, African Americans tended to have the highest numbers of partners, while among female subjects, Hispanic women had the fewest partners.

High-risk behaviors were also related to number of sexual partners. Being married or in a live-in relationship was associated with lower numbers of partners. For male subjects, alcohol use was predictive of higher numbers of partners. This finding did not hold true for females. Injection drug use was related to higher numbers of partners, with users of cocaine by injection having the highest number of partners. Having sex while being high was a predictor of higher numbers of sexual partners for men and women. For women, but not for men, exchanging sex for money was predictive of high numbers of partners.

Longshore and Anglin (1995) suggest modifying intervention strategies based on the finding that crack use is predictive of risk for both men and women. They point out that, in the past, intervention efforts in Los Angeles have been primarily directed at those who inject drugs, sexual partners of injection drug users, and women who offer sex for money. They suggest that future efforts may be more effective if they are directed at male and female crack users.

Poverty and Lack of Opportunity

Those living in poverty are at risk for many dangers and hardships. In this section, we examine the devastating effects of life in inner cities and homelessness in relation to unsafe sexual practices.

Susser and Gonzalez (1992) studied life in a New York City homeless shelter for men. These authors stress that the homeless are at very high risk for HIV infection because of their lack of permanent connection to others. They tend to have sexual relations with higher numbers of partners and have little access to knowledge about a partner's sexual history and the likelihood of associated risk. Residents of the shelter engaged in sex with each other in exchange for money. Women from outside the shelter engaged in sex with men from the shelter for money or drugs. Susser and Gonzalez found that sexual risk was compounded by the dangers associated with drug use. Thirty-eight percent of the residents of the shelter had current drug use or prior drug histories. Between 1988 and 1989, injected cocaine was the most frequently used drug for this population, raising concerns about HIV risk related to reused and shared needles.

AIDS prevention efforts were virtually nonexistent in the shelter before the study was initiated. When the level of knowledge of shelter residents was assessed, most had some knowledge of AIDS, but misinformation was common. Many residents felt that they were not at risk for contracting HIV. Some of the men believed that it was possible to determine another person's HIV status by his or her appearance, linking a lack of cleanliness or poor grooming with high likelihood for being HIV positive.

Obtaining conventional employment was difficult for shelter residents, and those who were interested and motivated to do so faced dealing with the stigma and inconvenience of being homeless when applying for a job. Susser and Gonzalez (1992) describe a series of challenges faced by one young man who wanted to find employment. He had difficulty actually producing a resume, had concerns about giving the address of the homeless shelter as his place of residence, and had problems coming up with references and proper attire. Many of the men chose less demanding and less legitimate ways of earning money, including begging and drug trafficking.

The hopelessness that exists for youth living in inner cities has been described by Bowser, Fullilove, and Fullilove (1990). Because their communities are economically devastated, offering very limited opportunities for decent incomes, and because the sale of drugs is their only viable financial opportunity, young people readily become drawn into this way of life. The risky sexual behavior that so often accompanies drug use is compounded by the perception of having no reason to postpone sexual activity until a later age. For example, Garbarino (1995) found that many such youth do not even expect to live to age 30. These adolescents become trapped into a very dangerous way of life that is difficult to escape. (See Chapter 4 for further discussion of interventions with this population.)

Post Traumatic Stress Disorder (PTSD) is a disorder caused by having one's life or personal safety threatened or by experiencing another person's exposure to such a threat, resulting in extreme fear accompanied by avoidance of situations that remind one of the trauma, heightened levels of arousal, and the tendency to relive the traumatic event (e.g., through flashbacks or nightmares, or in the case of children, through repetitive play associated with the trauma; American Psychiatric Association, 1994). PTSD is also a consequence of living under the harsh conditions of poverty described above (Garbarino, 1995). PTSD has been found to be related to one's parents having experienced poverty as well (Davidson, Hughes, Blazer, & George, 1991). Other predictors of PTSD include a history of child abuse, family members with psychological problems, and divorce of parents early in one's life.

Interpersonal Violence and Coercive Behavior

Sexual coercion ranges from verbal intimidation of a partner concerning safe sex practices to the use of physical force in sexual relationships. Biglan and colleagues (Biglan et al., 1995) examined the range of coercive sexual behaviors and found that substantial percentages from samples with presumably different levels of risk had experienced forced sex at some point. The percentage for college women was 22 percent, while 68 percent of adolescents who were homeless had been forced to have sex. Likewise, women in their study sometimes engaged in high-risk sexual behaviors, such as having sex without using a condom, because of pressure to do so from a partner. (For a more in-depth discussion of this study, see Chapter 5.)

As Biglan et al. (1995) found, sexual coercion can be a serious problem even in high-functioning college populations. In a study of attitudes about coercive sex, Sandberg, Jackson, and Petretic-Jackson (1987) found that 21 percent of their female subjects reported having been forced to have sex and 10 percent reported having been physically assaulted by a romantic partner. The male subjects in the study reported much lower rates of perpetrating sexual and physical abuse toward women, 2 percent and 1 percent, respectively. Women in the study were more likely than men to report that they had had sex when they did not wish to do so because they were reluctant to refuse their partner's request.

Another study of sexual coercion among college students included 472 men and 323 women (Miller & Marshall, 1987). Fifteen percent of the women in the sample reported having had sex when they did not want to do so because they believed their partners were too highly aroused to stop their behavior. Two percent of the women reported having been forced to have sex. More than half of the women who had been in a sexually coercive situation cited drug or alcohol use as a concomitant factor. The risk of having unprotected sex and consequently the risk of contracting HIV or other STDs in such situations is likely to be even higher than in cases when couples engage in consensual sex.

SUMMARY AND CONCLUSIONS

High-risk sexual behavior is influenced by many factors. In this chapter, we have discussed how a history of child maltreatment seems to be a particularly powerful predictor because of the increased likelihood of revictimization that results from dissociation. We also discussed how other related psychological factors such as denial and poor self-esteem play a role. Because the effects of child maltreatment are often linked to other behaviors that place individuals at risk, treatment for trauma is often an important component of effective interventions.

The use of alcohol and other drugs in relation to high-risk sexual behavior was examined. These substances may increase the risk of unsafe sex by decreasing inhibitions and impairing judgment. Injection drug use poses a threat to the users' sexual partners as well. Crack use is associated with very high risk for HIV infection. Therefore, treatment of substance abuse may play a critical role in reducing high-risk sexual behavior for some individuals.

Other problems, such as poverty and its consequences, have been presented, including the perception that for those in extreme poverty, there may seem to be no reason to postpone sexual activity. The homeless face particularly high risks because of the anonymity of their sexual encounters. Sexual coercion varies in its forms, ranging from the use of physical force to verbal intimidation. Risk increases for the victims in any case. Education remains an important priority, both for the purpose of informing those at risk and for convincing them of the level of risk that they actually face.

3

Models of Prevention

In this chapter, four specific, powerful models of prevention currently in use are presented, together with the effective intervention strategies that have developed out of these models. First, underlying theoretical concepts are described. Prochaska and DiClemente (1984) have delineated a five-stage model as a transtheoretical approach to understanding how human beings change behavior. The five stages (precontemplation, contemplation, preparation, action, and maintenance) are described here, along with the implications of this model for changing high-risk sexual behavior. Other cognitive behavioral constructs are then described which have been shown to be effective in designing effective intervention strategies, including the Theory of Reasoned Action (Azjen & Fishbein, 1980) and the Information-Motivation-Behavioral Skills (IMB) Model developed by Fisher and Fisher (1992) specifically for HIV prevention work. Various applications of the IMB Model are described, including the use of Natural Opinion Leaders (NOLs; Kelly et al., 1991) who generate support for the intervention among their peers. Next, "Reducing the Risk," a school-based intervention to decrease high-risk sexual behavior (Kirby, Barth, Leland, & Fetro, 1991), is described. Models for preventing teen pregnancy are then discussed, which include attention to the effects of personality factors, cognitive components, and social and environmental elements. Examples of interventions with teens in a clinic setting for pregnancy prevention, in a school environment with adolescent mothers, and in a multisite program for pregnant teens are described. We conclude with a summation of what we know so far about what is effective, and what is not, in this relatively young field of research.

Although the prevention field is relatively new and no one intervention has been designed that perfectly fits every circumstance or population, investigators have studied the components of risky behavior and examined elements required to change such behavior. Results of these studies have begun to shape the design of specific intervention programs. For example, education was once believed to be key to effective intervention, but research has indicated that education alone is rarely successful (Shoop & Davidson, 1994). On the one hand, studies have demonstrated that, within high-risk populations, there are large gaps in knowledge of transmission of HIV and other STDs, and a strong tendency to endorse many myths and fallacies about these diseases (Sweat & Levin, 1995). Yet, even where knowledge of transmission is fairly accurate (e.g., among college students), individuals engage in risky behavior and fail to protect themselves, perhaps because of a failure to perceive themselves as at risk (Shoop & Davidson, 1994; Rotheram-Borus and Koopman, 1991; Wulfert & Wan, 1993).

Consequently, slogans such as "Just Say No" rarely achieve the goals for which they were designed. Education programs must be carried out in conjunction with other approaches designed to impact the environment of the group selected. These multifaceted approaches must include an emphasis on increasing knowledge, social support, and competency of the individual, while also producing changes in the larger social structure. Attention to cultural diversity, so that materials are presented in a manner relevant to the understanding and norms of the targeted group, is essential (considerations for interventions with specific ethnic groups are discussed at length in chapter 4). Developmental factors also must be given attention, so that appropriate levels of cognitive awareness are utilized (Wells et al., 1995; Hoppe, Wells, Wilsdon, Gillmore, & Morrison, 1994).

In their review article of 1994, Choi and Coates examined studies of high-risk populations, including gay and bisexual men, injection drug users, commercial sex workers, patients of STD clinics, young adults (age 18 to 29), adolescents, and adult heterosexuals. Across the studies of these populations, they found that many AIDS prevention programs had been shown to be effective in producing long-term changes in risky sexual behavior (in 20 out of 77 studies, or 26 percent).

In fact, with effective interventions such as those discussed in this chapter, dramatic changes in sexual behavior have been accomplished in some groups in a relatively short period of time. Coates (1990) reported that, among a sample of gay men in San Francisco, unprotected anal intercourse dropped within a three-year period in the 1980s from 33.9 percent (receptive) and 37.4 percent (insertive) to 4.2 and 1.7 percent, respectively.

A BROAD MODEL FOR PREVENTION: STAGES OF BEHAVIORAL CHANGE

Prochaska, DiClemente, and colleagues (Prochaska & DiClemente, 1982; Prochaska, DiClemente, & Norcross, 1992) have proposed a five-stage model of human change, which they have found useful in predicting and enhancing the ability of individuals to make changes in problem behaviors. In searching for principles to all types of change, Prochaska and DiClemente focused specifically on intentional change. They developed a transtheoretical approach which is designed to account for both self-initiated changes and professionally assisted change (e.g., psychotherapy).

The five-stage model they developed has been shown in numerous studies to be effective in explaining change across a variety of problem behaviors (e.g., smoking, diet, chemical dependency, safer sex, and condom use). The five stages of the model are described briefly below (Prochaska, DiClemente, & Norcross, 1992).

Stage 1. Precontemplation

The first stage is that of *precontemplation*, described as a period in which individuals engage in risky behavior with little or no awareness of the consequences. At this stage, there is typically not even a recognition of the problem, although others close to the individual may be well aware of the problem. The alcoholic in denial is a classic example of an individual in precontemplation, where the family may be telling the person he or she needs to change, but he or she is vehemently opposed to the suggestion. Some in precontemplation may have a notion that the behavior is a potential problem, but the key feature of this stage is an unwillingness to acknowledge the problem or to consider what might be required to change it.

Prochaska (1994) reports that at least 50 percent of those at risk because of behavior problems are in the precontemplation stage, with no intention of taking any action (estimates from studies range from 40 to 80 percent, depending on the population studied). Consequently, it is imperative that we learn more about what motivates individuals to move from precontemplation to the next phase of change, *contemplation*.

Stage 2. Contemplation

The contemplation stage is marked by an awareness of the need to change a particular behavior, yet without the commitment to action that would be required to actually make changes. Contemplation may last for years, Prochaska and DiClemente (1984) have found. This stage is marked by serious consideration of the payoffs and costs of the problematic behavior.

To continue with the example of alcoholism, individuals may move into contemplation when something in the environment shifts dramatically because of their drinking: e.g., they are fired or their spouse leaves, or they have a car accident while intoxicated. Such outside forces may only be sufficient to bring the problem into their conscious awareness, yet in the five-stage model, this is considered a step toward change. In contemplation, the alcoholic continues to drink, but begins to be aware of a variety of consequences, such as the hungover feeling each morning, the fights with loved ones about the drinking, or the risks of driving under the influence. Although they take no action, individuals at this stage are considering action as a possibility.

Stage 3. Preparation

In the preparation stage, individuals have not previously taken any successful action toward changing the problem behavior, but they have made definite plans to begin in the near future. They may have attempted to decrease the behavior; for example, the alcoholic is consuming fewer drinks each day, or he or she may switch from hard liquor to beer, in an attempt to decrease alcohol consumption. The action at this stage is relatively ineffective, however; rather, it serves to mark the beginning stages of action. For this reason, some researchers conceptualize this stage as an early phase of the action stage. Prochaska and his colleagues earlier termed it decision-making, but have now returned to the use of their earlier term, preparation (Prochaska, DiClemente, & Norcross, 1992).

Stage 4. Action

Being in the action phase of change is defined as having successfully modified the behavior for a time period of one day to six months. In other words, individuals have made a commitment to change their behavior, and they are taking actions consistent with that commitment. Conceptualizing this as a stage of change, rather than an end point, has allowed for the recognition that commitment and action alone are insufficient to permanently alter a behavior. At the same time, it also allows for the understanding that short-term changes, otherwise known as relapse behaviors, do not reflect a lack of commitment to change, but rather are part and parcel of the process of change.

Thus, during the action stage the alcoholic may begin to attend Alcoholics Anonymous, may stop drinking for a few days at a time, and may substantially reduce the volume of alcohol consumed. Repeatedly falling back into the behavior is expected and predictable, and thus can be managed through specific intervention techniques, such as relapse prevention strategies (Curtin, Stephens, & Roffman, 1997; deWit & van Griensven, 1994). Being in action means frequently returning to the saddle after falling off the horse, practicing the behaviors necessary for change until they become habitual.

Stage 5. Maintenance

Once behavior changes have become successfully incorporated into the individual's life for at least six months, the individual is considered to be in the maintenance stage of change. For addictive behaviors, maintenance may be a stage that lasts a lifetime, during which relapse-prevention behaviors are continuously practiced.

For example, the alcoholic with six months of sobriety in AA receives a coin and recognition for this hallmark of change (as well as at the one month, three month, and yearly intervals). Changes may still be quite fragile at this point, so that the individual may continue to need a considerable amount of support for months or even years. Maintenance is marked by stabilization of changes and work on relapse avoidance.

Recycling through the Stages

Work with addictive behavior allowed Prochaska and colleagues (Prochaska, DiClemente, & Norcross, 1992) to recognize that many individuals may relapse in such a way that they drop back to earlier stages of change. That is, individuals in action who relapse with alcohol or smoking may feel they have failed, or that they are incapable of changing the behavior. These individuals may return to contemplation or preparation, or even back to precontemplation. The authors report that as many as 15 percent of relapsers may return to precontemplation, but that 85 percent return to later stages, and frequently these individuals recycle to a higher stage than they did at earlier relapses. Thus, recycling back through the stages of change should be considered a normative experience that is part of the process of changing a behavior that is firmly entrenched.

Targeting Interventions to Change Phase

Research has been conducted to apply the theoretical stages of change model to a host of human behavior problems, most with implications for health and human safety for the individual and for others around them (e.g., addictions, delinquency). One specific study by Prochaska et al. (1994) examined the model's application to 12 problem behaviors, to determine differences and similarities related to stages of change and decisional balance.

The 12 behavior changes included: (1) practicing safer sex, (2) using condoms, (3) quitting smoking, (4) ceasing cocaine use, (5) controlling weight, (6) reducing dietary fat, (7) decreasing youth delinquency behaviors, (8) applying sunscreen, (9) testing for radon gas, (10) exercising, (11) obtaining a mammography exam, and (12) physicians practicing intervention techniques with patients who smoke. For the study of safer sex practices, subjects were 213 sexually active college students recruited from college classrooms who were predominantly white (96 percent), female (79 percent), and single (94 percent). Subjects for the condom-use study were 345 men and women with histories of high-risk sexual behavior, recruited through street interviews and newspaper ads; samples within this group were studied at different stages of change. Mean ages for each stage's sample in the condom-use study ranged from 29.4 years (action stage) to 33 years (precontemplation stage). The ethnic composition of the total condom-use sample was 50 percent Caucasian, 36.5 percent African American, 12 percent Hispanic, 1 percent Native American, and 0.5 percent Asian.

Across the 12 problem behaviors, strong similarities were observed in relation to the stages of change (Prochaska et al., 1994). The study demonstrated that a simple two-factor solution accounted for differences in stages of change. The perception by the individual of the pros and cons for the behavior was found to be the best predictor of stages of change. That is, across all 12 behaviors, the perceived costs of changing the behavior were greater than the perceived benefits of change for individuals in the precontemplation stage. In the action stage, however, the payoffs of changing were perceived as greater than the costs of continuing the behavior for 11 of the 12 problems, including safer sex practices and condom use (cocaine use was the exception, but this sample was confounded by residency in treatment programs at the time of the study).

For seven of the 12 problems (including the two related to sexual practices), benefits of change began to outweigh the costs of making the change during the stage of contemplation. With the remaining behaviors (delinquency, sunscreen, high-fat diet, mammography), the crossover from viewing change as a cost to seeing it as a payoff appeared during the action phase (with the exception of exercise, where the crossover occurred during the stage of preparation). However, Prochaska et al. (1994) suggested that crossover appearing in the action stage may actually reflect a shift that occurred during the preparation phase for these five behaviors.

Implications of these findings are that, in the early stages of change, individuals benefit from boosts to their positive motivation for change. Thus, increasing their perception of the benefits of changing the behavior is most likely to move them from precontemplation into contemplation. However, Prochaska et al. (1994) further suggest that once the individual moves into contemplation, work at decreasing their perceptions of the costs of the change may help to continue their progress toward the action and maintenance phases of change.

Stages of Change Applied to High-Risk Sexual Behavior

In addition to the study described above of 12 risky behaviors (which included condom use and high-risk sexual activity), at least one other study has attempted to apply the transtheoretical model to interventions with risky sexual behavior (Grimley, Riley, Bellis, & Prochaska, 1993). Grimley and colleagues examined contraceptive behaviors as they related to pregnancy and disease prevention. Initially, they developed measures to study decisional balance (i.e., payoffs versus costs) in choosing to use or not to use contraceptives. These instruments provided information regarding where each subject was in regard to positive motivation (PROS) and negative attributions (CONS) about using contraception.

In this sample of heterosexual college students, 72 percent reported using a birth control method every time they had sex, with 28 percent reporting inconsistent use of birth control. Participants were then assessed for their stage of change. Although only 6.4 percent were in the precontemplation stage regarding pregnancy prevention, the more significant finding was that 63.6 percent of these young students did not consistently use condoms for prevention of STDs. In fact, a full 37.4 percent were in precontemplation about the use of condoms, indicating they had no plans to begin using them anytime in the future.

Thus, Grimley et al. (1993) concluded that these college students were much further in the stage of change model with regard to pregnancy prevention than they were for prevention of STDs. The authors concluded that, if prevention efforts are to be effective, they must address individual perspectives on risky behavior. Individuals in this group do not clearly perceive themselves to be at risk for STDs.

Specific recommendations included strong messages designed to emphasize the positive reasons for changing behavior (PROS), as this was the weakest area for individuals who were in the precontemplation stage regarding condom use and pregnancy prevention. The authors suggest the use of consciousness raising and self-reevaluation strategies to increase the perception of the advantages, or PROS (e.g., protection from pregnancy and disease, ease of use, availability), of engaging in healthy behavior for individuals within the target group. This finding is in line with the findings from the Prochaska et al. (1994) study, described above, which indicated that increasing the positive motivation was the best way to move individuals from precontemplation into contemplation.

SPECIFIC MODELS FOR PREVENTING HIGH-RISK SEXUAL BEHAVIOR

Theory of Reasoned Action

In attempting to describe and understand sexual behavior, many researchers have used the Theory of Reasoned Action (Azjen & Fishbein, 1980). This theory states that individual behavior is most effectively predicted by the person's intention to engage in a particular action. Reasoned action theory proposes that the potential for behaviors to be adopted is a function of their being highly valued or seen as desirable to the individual, as well as within the normative peer group. Related to sexual behavior, the choice to modify one's behavior occurs within a context of the perception and value placed on the prevention behaviors in question. That is, engaging in safer sex will depend upon the degree to which the individual sees it as necessary and desirable to him- or herself, and perceives these practices as being acceptable to and valued by members of the individual's peer group.

Using the Theory of Reasoned Action (Azjen & Fishbein, 1980), researchers have attempted to gain a better understanding of sexual behavior and the decision-making related to it. In one study of adolescents, Kegeles, Adler, and Irwin (1988) found that exposure to information about AIDS had little effect on the teens' behavior, just as findings noted earlier in this chapter indicated education alone is insufficient to change behavior. These youth reported that they believed condoms protect against STDs and that such protection is valuable. Yet both genders reported a lack of intention to use condoms or to encourage their partners to use them. After the educational presentation, males actually showed some decline in intentionality. Their decision-making processes were more strongly linked to broader social expectations and to more general attitudes than to specific beliefs about AIDS.

Likewise, Weisman et al. (1991) assessed 408 adolescent girls' (age 11 to 18) contraceptive decision-making using the Theory of Reasoned Action. The teens' perceived risk did not predict their use of condoms at the last reported sexual encounter; rather, the greatest predictor of condom use was having asked a partner to use a condom in the past. These findings suggest girls may have a greater impact on prevention for both genders than has often been assumed. Other researchers have reported similar findings of a relationship between willingness to ask partners to use condoms and greater frequency of condom use (Catania et al., 1989).

Information-Motivation-Behavioral Skills Model

The Information-Motivation-Behavioral Skills (IMB) model was developed by Fisher and Fisher (1992) specifically for work with HIV prevention, initially in the college population. The IMB Model suggests that whether individuals engage in preventive behaviors during sex is fundamentally determined by their level of information (i.e., knowledge), their motivation, and their behavioral skills.

Specifically, the first step toward prevention is the individual acquisition of accurate information regarding HIV transmission and its prevention. Beyond that, motivation to avoid risk and to engage in preventive behaviors will include personal motives (such as fear of becoming sick or positive attitudes toward preventive behaviors), social motivation (e.g., one's peers also endorse and engage in prevention), and the individual perception that one is personally vulnerable to being infected. The third determinant of preventive behavior is the individual's level of behavioral skills. This factor allows him or her to engage in the preventive activity and includes the assertiveness necessary to ask a partner to accept preventive methods, the knowledge of how to use preventive measures (e.g., condoms), the expectation that he or she will be successful in obtaining the partner's agreement, and the expectation that he or she will be able to correctly use protective measures (i.e., a sense of self-efficacy regarding engaging in protective behaviors).

Fisher and Fisher (1992) propose that information and motivation to engage in HIV prevention are expressed through the individual's behavioral skills, which in turn affect the degree to which prevention activity is begun and maintained. That is, level of information and motivation to engage in prevention are only as effective as the individual's ability to carry them out through the negotiation of a social situation. Thus, the behavioral skills are a key element, for they have the ability to set limits on the effects of the other two factors in the model.

Furthermore, an individual may have requisite skills necessary to engage in prevention under most circumstances, but situations may arise which require negotiations for which they have no information, training, or skill development (e.g., coercion or force). Fisher and colleagues describe information and motivation as independent constructs in the IMB model for HIV prevention (Fisher, Fisher, Williams, & Malloy, 1994).

IMB Model: Applications

The IMB model was described and developed under a five-year grant from the National Institutes for Mental Health (NIMH). During that period, Fisher and Fisher (1992, 1993) tested the hypothesized relationships within the model and their application to prevention of HIV transmission. These relationships were confirmed with culturally diverse high school populations. The model has been tested with high-risk populations to determine which factors are most relevant to engaging in risky sexual behavior and their fit with the model. Studies with university populations have demonstrated the model's usefulness in successful interventions to increase prevention behaviors. The model is unique for its thorough specification and empirical validation of constructs and their applicability to populations at risk for HIV transmission.

Once their studies had documented the validity of the IMB model for HIV prevention (e.g., constructs of the model explained 55 percent of the variance in prevention behavior among multiracial high school students), Fisher and Fisher (1995) began to develop the applications aspects of the IMB model. Using an approach known as elicitation research, they conducted studies to uncover the deficits in information, motivation, and behavioral skills that are relevant to HIV prevention for specific populations. Elicitation research involves techniques such as questionnaires and focus groups, which provide information that allows for interventions targeted to specific populations, addressing the particular needs of that group. Evaluation research is then conducted as the intervention is delivered, to ensure that the targeted changes are actually realized.

Elicitation research has been conducted with samples of gay male adults, heterosexual adults, heterosexual college students, and with (predominantly heterosexual) multiracial high school students (Fisher & Fisher, 1995). Below are some of the research findings for each portion of the model.

Information

In a sample of 1255 multiracial high school students in Miami, early findings from brief questionnaires have revealed significant deficits in HIV transmission knowledge (e.g., most were not able to differentiate the relatively lower risk of oral sex compared to sexual intercourse, and many believed HIV could be transmitted through saliva). Deficits were also apparent in the students' judgment regarding a partner's HIV status. Students tended to endorse beliefs that indicated they could determine a partner was HIV negative based on appearance, acquaintance with the individual, or some other judgment of the individual's personality, status, or life situation. These faulty judgments have been determined to be a key element in the prediction of high-risk sexual behavior.

Motivation

The Miami sample also revealed important motivational deficits among these high school students (Fisher & Fisher, 1995). A majority of sexually active students reported doubts that their sexual partners would want to use condoms and doubts that their friends were using them; this was particularly true for males. Similar findings were reported for a sample of 357 multiracial ninth graders from Worcester, Massachusetts. In addition to the findings about social pressure, the Miami results regarding internal attitudes revealed most students believed condoms interfered with sexual pleasure, and most of the sexually active students of both genders believed their risk of HIV infection was below average to no risk of infection.

Behavioral Skills

In the Miami sample, less than half reported they felt confident they could refuse to have unsafe sex in a specific situation; in the Worcester sample, 56 percent reported they would have difficulty abstaining from sexual intercourse (Fisher & Fisher, 1995). Furthermore, about half of the Miami students reported being sexually active, but less than half of the sexually active group reported consistent condom use. With new partners in the prior year, 49 percent of the students had had discussions about safer sex practices. Less than a third (27 percent) of the students who had been in a situation with the possibility of unsafe sex reported they had consistently refused to engage in it. Fisher and Fisher note that these findings are similar to those reported by other researchers in the field.

From focus group work with college students (primarily heterosexual), Fisher and Fisher (1995) report this population has misconceptions similar to those found among high school students. That is, they make judgments about a partner's risk based on unreliable criteria such as personality factors, their closeness to the partner, their belief that the relationship is monogamous, and other variables related to the partner's status, traits, and outward appearance. Furthermore, many believe that introducing safer sex practices would threaten the relationship with their partner, as well. As in the high school sample, college students were not particularly motivated to practice safe sex, they had faulty views of themselves as having little or no risk of infection, and they viewed condoms as unpleasant and as interfering with sexual enjoyment. Particularly significant was the finding that few students felt confident that they could negotiate with a partner regarding condom use.

Based on these findings, Fisher and Fisher (1995) suggest that the negotiation model which has often been used in teaching safe sex practices does not work well in actual situations. Students reported many instances where they felt unable or ineffective in attempting negotiations (e.g., before sexual desire has been verbalized in a relationship, when intoxicated, or in high sexual arousal states). Reports from the college students indicated brief, "one-liner," or highly directive statements were most likely to be effective strategies to teach these young adults (e.g., "put this on," "you bring the wine, I'll bring the condoms," Fisher & Fisher, 1995, p. 10).

Further development of effective interventions is currently underway, through Fisher and Fisher's (1995) NIMH grant to continue the elicitation research, as well as conduct the delivery and evaluation of interventions with multiracial high school students in New England. The intervention includes the use of teaching videos which depict young people in situations relevant to the audience, discussing safe sex practices or applying them, and also of young people who are HIV positive talking about their own situation and how their lack of knowledge and their faulty assumptions put them at risk. In addition to the IMB model, the interventions will incorporate the effective intervention strategy of utilizing peer "Natural Opinion Leaders" (NOLs; described below) to impact group norms by enlisting the support of the leaders within the targeted peer group. Developed by Kelly and associates (Kelly et al., 1991, 1992), the NOL model has proven to be highly effective in changing behavior related to HIV prevention. By combining the empirically validated IMB model with the NOL model, Fisher and Fisher's intervention with high school students is expected to be highly effective.

Natural Opinion Leaders

Kelly and colleagues (Kelly et al., 1991) developed an AIDS prevention strategy based on the use of peer leaders who endorse desired changes. This strategy was tested to determine whether such leadership endorsements would create or speed up behavior changes in a larger population to decrease risk of HIV infection. Employing 43 opinion leaders who were popular among their gay peers in a small city, researchers trained the leaders to make endorsements for changing the target behavior. The selected city was compared to two comparison cities at two baseline periods (Total N = 659) and at two postintervention periods (Total N = 608). In a two-month period, gay men in the intervention city reported rates of unprotected anal intercourse which decreased from 36.9 percent to 27.5 percent; they reported a 16 percent increase in condom use during anal intercourse, and there was an 18 percent decline in the numbers of men who reported multiple sex partners. Comparison cities showed no significant changes in sexual behavior among control subjects.

A similar intervention used a group of popular "trendsetters" identified by bartenders in three small cities (Kelly et al., 1992). These opinion leaders endorsed behavior changes with gay male peers in the different cities. The trendsetters were trained in peer education, communication of suggestions, and endorsement of risk-reduction behaviors. The intervention was introduced sequentially in each city with a lag time between each introduction. Surveys pre- and postintervention revealed systematic reductions in high-risk behavior (e.g., unprotected anal intercourse reduced from 15 to 29 percent from baseline), which were replicated across all three cities.

Furthermore, this work has been extended to demonstrate that educational videotapes presenting AIDS prevention information were significantly more effective with African-American urban women when the taped presenters were also African-American women (Kalichman, Kelly, Hunter, Murphy & Tyler, 1993). Participants who saw tapes of ethnically and culturally matched presenters were significantly more likely to have discussed AIDS with friends, to be more sensitized to AIDS risk, to have been tested for HIV, and to ask for condoms at the follow-up than were those not seeing a matched video.

"Reducing the Risk": A School-Based Intervention

"Reducing the Risk" is a sex education curriculum designed to decrease high-risk sexual practices among California high school students (Kirby et al., 1991), introduced into 13 California high schools, with 758 high school students assigned to either treatment or control groups. The authors note that this intervention is an outgrowth of earlier attempts at changing sexual behavior patterns of adolescents. This later generation approach capitalizes on lessons learned from earlier efforts, makes use of theoretical constructs found helpful for other health issues (e.g., substance abuse), and includes an evaluation component which is methodologically rigorous.

Based on a combination of social learning theory, social inoculation theory, and cognitive behavioral theory (Bandura, 1986), the curriculum uses teachers and peers who model the desired behavior and then ask students to practice these behaviors through role-playing (Kirby et al., 1991). Thus, the intervention includes elements of education, social support, and the development of specific competencies. Social pressures for sexual activity are discussed, along with the typical conversations common to this type of pressure. Students are taught to resist and practice resisting this pressure with verbal strategies, including talking about abstinence and birth control. Over time, the scenarios presented increase in difficulty, and the students require less assistance in responding as they gain more confidence in their ability to resist pressure. Finally, the curriculum teaches social skills which help students apply their newly acquired knowledge about safer sex and pregnancy prevention, and also gives them practice in obtaining relevant information from clinics and drug stores.

Participants in the "Reducing the Risk" curriculum were assessed before the intervention, immediately after, and at six months and 18 months after exposure to the curriculum. Findings from this study indicated that students who were not yet sexually active at the onset benefited most from the intervention. That is, these students were significantly less likely to have become sexually active at the 18-month follow-up, and if they did become sexually active, they were significantly less likely to engage in unprotected sex than control subjects who were not sexually active at the beginning (Kirby et al., 1991). For students who were already sexually active at the onset of the program, however, the curriculum had no effects on frequency of sexual intercourse or on use of contraceptives. For all participants, the program significantly increased students' knowledge and their communication with parents about issues of abstinence and contraception. Finally, the positive effects for the treatment group not sexually active at onset were found across subgroups, including Latinos, whites, low-risk, and high-risk youth; these findings were especially strong for the lower risk teens and for females.

MODELS FOR PREVENTING TEEN PREGNANCY

Theoretical models for teen pregnancy prevention overlap those for prevention of STDs, despite some differences in the issues involved. Rickel (1989) outlined four broad approaches to understanding why adolescents become pregnant: (1) ignorance of contraception; (2) personality variables; (3) cognitive models; and (4) social and environmental factors. Contraceptive ignorance has found the least support in controlled studies, a finding complementary to HIV-prevention research, cited earlier, which indicated education alone does not change behavior (Shoop & Davidson, 1994).

Personality Factors

Personality variables, on the other hand, have been implicated as significant in distinguishing pregnant/parenting teens from their peers. Thomas and Rickel (1995), comparing 420 high school students' scores on the Minnesota Multiphasic Personality Inventory (MMPI), found significantly more maladjustment among the 179 pregnant or parenting teens within the sample. Of these girls, 79 percent scored in the clinical range on the MMPI, compared to just 21 percent of the nonpregnant/nonparenting controls in the sample. Furthermore, a discriminate function analysis using MMPI scores correctly differentiated 80 percent of the full sample of 420 students as pregnant/parenting or control teens (p < .001).

Based on this study and other ongoing research, Becker-Lausen and Rickel (1995) proposed a model (see Figure 2.1) suggesting that elevated MMPI profiles reflected symptoms of trauma in these adolescents. Initial studies testing the model have supported this proposition, suggesting a mechanism by which negative outcomes are transmitted from generation to generation (Rickel & Becker, 1997).

Cognitive Aspects

Cognitive models, such as those described above for preventing STDs, have also been applied to teen pregnancy prevention. For example, Adler (1994) combines motivation and decision-making variables with psychosocial factors affecting adolescents. She notes that teens, just like adults, underestimate the risks of getting pregnant or contracting an STD. This does not result from a deficiency in the teen, Adler suggests, but rather because teens, like all human beings, are "optimistically biased" when an outcome is indefinite (p. 4). That is, most people believe their personal likelihood of being the victim of a bad event, whether it is a car accident, illness, crime, or unplanned pregnancy, is less than the actual risk for the average person. In fact, research has indicated adolescents are no more optimistically biased than adults, Adler notes, despite the belief that teens are inclined to see themselves as invulnerable.

In controlled, long-term studies of adolescent behavior, Adler (1994) found a significant relationship between stated intention to use specific methods of contraception and their actual use, even when subjects changed partners during the time period examined. Furthermore, beliefs were found to be important predictors of intention to use specific forms of contraception. For example, intention to use condoms was found to be associated with different beliefs for males and females, after controlling for race/ethnicity, whether the teens were sexually active, and prior use of condoms.

For females, intention to use condoms was associated with beliefs that (1) use enabled sex on the spur of the moment; (2) condoms are easy to use; (3) use is popular with peers; (4) use requires a partner to have self-control; (5) condoms are clean; and (6) they have no side effects. For males, intention to use condoms was associated with beliefs that (1) condoms allow sex on the spur of the moment; (2) they are easy to use; (3) condoms are not painful to use; (4) they can be used without parents' knowledge; (5) condom use decreases guilt; and (6) condoms do not affect one's looks. The last finding surprised researchers, who had included this belief for women taking birth-control pills, who may feel they will gain weight or experience other appearance changes as a result of these hormones. Males' endorsement (in reverse), associated with condom use, indicated that some males may not use condoms because they believe they would look strange wearing them.

Finally, Adler (1994) found two essential beliefs that were not related to intention to use condoms for either males or females: (1) condoms prevent pregnancy; and (2) condoms prevent STDs. However, the lack of endorsement of these beliefs in this context did not mean adolescents did not *know* that condoms were capable of preventing these outcomes. Rather, knowing these facts had *no* effect on whether or not the adolescents personally intended to use them.

This finding is extremely important for prevention efforts, reminding us again of the importance of the value of reinforcement to the individual (Rotter, 1954/1980), and providing an explanation for the inadequacy of education alone to change behavior. Adler (1994) suggests knowledge of condom effectiveness for health outcomes is "a necessary but not sufficient condition for their use" (p. 10).

Social and Environmental Factors

Studies of pregnant teens have reported 30 to 60 percent of them say they wanted to become pregnant (Rickel, 1989). Among adolescents in general, about 20 percent indicate they see becoming pregnant as a positive outcome (Adler, 1994). Reviewing the findings related to pregnancy intention, Rickel (1989) suggested babies may represent hope or a hopeful future to some teens, or they may fill a teen's need for love, attachment, and affection. Pregnancy may gain attention for the adolescent, may be a rebellious act, or may be a means of gaining autonomy or adult status.

Adler (1994) noted that retrospective studies have linked teen pregnancy to low self-esteem and lower educational attainment; however, she reported that her prospective research indicated an interaction between these variables: ". . . those teens who are already doing poorly in school, have low self-esteem, and who do not see much chance of gaining esteem through academic performance appear to see pregnancy and motherhood as an alternative path" (p. 12). She concludes that becoming pregnant is a logical consequence of the expectation inherent in this view of motherhood, even though the reality of the experience may fail to meet the teens' expectations.

Beck and Davies (1987) reviewed the literature on programs designed to increase teen use of birth control, and they reported several themes that emerged from this literature: (1) Interventions which focus on teens' concerns, such as skill-building in communication and problem-solving, are the most effective; (2) programs which invite the involvement of the teens' significant others, without mandating it, appear to be promising; (3) studies of college populations have identified important emotional issues, such as guilt and anxiety, related to sexual behavior, yet little work has been done to examine this component of behavior for younger adolescents; (4) studies related to teen contraceptive use have tended to focus on female adolescents, neglecting the study of adolescent boys (other than college students).

Pregnancy Prevention Programs: Clinic-Based Services

The Family Health Council of Central Pennsylvania, representing 41 reproductive health clinics in a 24-county region, developed an experimental intervention designed to meet the specific needs of adolescents seeking family planning services (Winter & Breckenmaker, 1991). The intervention stressed in-depth counseling, developmentally appropriate education, reassurance, and social support. Education was provided one-on-one, using concrete concepts and visual aids.

Teenagers were scheduled for two appointments, one for counseling and education and the second for the medical examination, usually within two weeks of each other (Winter & Breckenmaker, 1991). The birth-control method was started after the second appointment; follow-up visits were scheduled for six weeks after the initial visit. All staff members were trained in adolescent psychosocial development; one staff member was designated and trained as the teen counselor. Participation of males was encouraged; parent and friend participation was also encouraged. However, the teen was assured of confidentiality rights and was always provided time alone with the counselor. Staff taught patients to recognize and resist peer pressure.

This experimental protocal was tested against the typical service delivery practices using 1261 predominantly white patients under age 18 at six nonmetropolitan family planning clinics (Winter & Breckenmaker, 1991). As random assignment was not feasible, the six sites were chosen for their equivalency in terms of socioeconomic status, ethnicity, and staffing patterns. Three sites were designated for the experimental intervention; three were used as controls. Pretest and posttest measures were administered to all subjects in three broad categories: (1) knowledge acquired by patients; (2) patients' feelings toward the clinic; and

(3) patients' family planning experiences, including use of contraceptives, clinic attendance, and incidence of unintended pregnancy.

Results of the comparison studies of control sites and intervention sites indicated those teens receiving the intervention services had significantly greater gains in their knowledge base and in their use of contraceptives six months after their initial visit (Winter & Breckenmaker, 1991). Adolescents who received the intervention services also had significantly fewer problems using contraceptives and significantly fewer pregnancies six months after their initial contact. In addition, teenagers at the experimental sites were less likely to have become pregnant a year after the initial visit than those at the control sites.

Investigators noted the study's limitations, primarily the lack of generalizability to nonwhite, urban populations, and recommended the protocal be tested with inner-city clinics serving these populations (Winter & Breckenmaker, 1991). Nevertheless, they concluded that "the investment of extra time and effort to address the nonmedical needs of adolescent family planning patients pays off . . . [helping] these patients use their methods successfully, continue using them despite problems, deal with problems more easily. . . . [H]owever, the emphasis on psychosocial needs seems to help patients avoid pregnancy, the bottom line of family planning service provision" (p. 30).

Interventions with Teen Mothers: School-Based Programs

Because a teen who has a second child soon after her first is at greatest risk for a life of poverty and disadvantage, many pregnancy prevention programs have focused on the already pregnant or parenting teen to support them in finishing school and delaying subsequent childbearing (Seitz & Apfel, 1993). One approach to this tertiary intervention strategy is a separate, alternative school for adolescent girls who are pregnant and/or parenting.

Seitz and Apfel (1993) followed a cohort of young mothers in such an alternative public school program in New Haven, Connecticut. Participants were adolescents who delivered their first-born infants between 1979 and 1980, who were less than 19 at delivery, and who had not yet graduated from high school when they became pregnant.

Researchers found that 87 percent of the teens who met this criteria were from low-income families, and thus, they chose to limit the study to that socioeconomic group. In addition, a large majority of teens in the school were African-American adolescents; therefore, the study was also limited to black teen mothers. The final study sample consisted of 102 black teenage mothers.

The subjects were enrolled in the alternative program at the Polly T. McCabe Center in New Haven, where the rules of attendance were similar to random assignment in determining the length of the postnatal intervention received (Seitz & Apfel, 1993). Thus, it was possible to compare those girls who were in the alternative program seven weeks or less to those who attended for more than seven weeks. The two groups were compared for confounding variables, but no significant differences were found between the groups on such factors as age at delivery, previous pregnancy, age at menarche, grades, school attendance, death of mother, or number of siblings. Researchers conducted extensive interviews with participants (as well as with their mothers) when the teens' infants were 18 months old. Follow-up data on subsequent births were gathered two years and five years after the first birth.

The Polly T. McCabe Center, a separate school for pregnant girls, is part of the New Haven public school system (Seitz & Apfel, 1993). In addition to regular classes, social and medical services are provided to pregnant teens. Staff include teachers, nurses, and social workers who are racially and ethnically diverse. Based on a family management approach, counseling is designed to help a pregnant or parenting student plan for her future by helping her deal with such issues as delaying pregnancy, finding day care, handling family conflict, finding housing, and staying in school. Counselors include nurses from Yale University's School of Nursing, who also teach the childbirth classes, and social workers from Yale-New Haven Hospital.

At the two-year and five-year evaluations, the two groups of teen mothers had significantly different birth rates for subsequent children; that is, those receiving longer than seven-week interventions at McCabe were significantly less likely to have had a second birth at either time period than those with shorter interventions (Seitz & Apfel, 1993). Specifically, within two years of the first birth, 19 of 52 (36 percent) students in the shorter program had delivered a second child, compared to 6 of 50 (12 percent) of those with the longer intervention.

At five years, three subjects had been lost to follow-up, and 35 of 50 (70 percent) of the young women in the shorter-term intervention had delivered one or more additional children, whereas 22 of 49 (45 percent) who received the longer program had additional children. All of these differences were statistically significant; they did not change when researchers controlled for infertility, miscarriages, and abortions. Furthermore, the delay of additional children was found to have significant, beneficial effects on the mothers' educational attainment and welfare dependency.

Seitz and Apfel (1993) suggest, based on these findings, that a critical period exists in the second month following the birth of the first child during which a teen mother may make decisions which have ramifications for the course of the rest of her life. This period coincides with the time when sexual activity is most likely to resume, after healing has occurred postpartum. The authors suggest that provision of a support structure during this critical time may be essential to the mother's ability to make decisions which will ensure she and her infant have the best possible future.

Ounce of Prevention: Multisite Interventions for Pregnant Teens

The Ounce of Prevention Fund (OPF) is a network of programs sponsored by the Illinois Department of Children and Family Services. Based on a family support and education model, OPF programs are conducted in a variety of settings, including medical clinics, child welfare agencies, child care centers, and family support centers. OPF has a statewide adolescent pregnancy project known as Parents Too Soon, which was the focus of evaluation research conducted by Ruch-Ross, Jones, and Musick (1992).

OPF closely monitors and provides technical assistance to programs to ensure uniformity of service delivery (Ruch-Ross et al., 1992). The programs offer home visiting, as well as weekly education and support groups for parents. For teens in this study sample, home visiting and parent support groups were the predominant interventions. Goals of the programs included delaying subsequent pregnancies and fostering economic independence.

Home visitors in these programs were paraprofessionals trained by OPF and local sites to help reduce the isolation of teen mothers, to link them to community resources, and to provide home-based information and support. Home visitation is an intervention originally developed using professional nurses as home visitors, which has been shown in empirical studies to be effective in improving the health and development of women and their children (Kitzman, Cole, Yoos, & Olds, 1997). The use of paraprofessionals as home visitors is a newer development (Hiatt, Sampson, & Baird, 1997), which has the potential benefit of visitors as powerful role models with whom clients can readily identify, and visitors who may feel greater empathy for the clients because of closer identification with their issues and problems.

Parent support groups in the OPF programs operated on a peer support model and were led by trained facilitators. Most facilitators had been teen mothers themselves. They educated the teen mothers about child health and development while also providing emotional support. Parent support models have been promoted as a means of parents helping parents with a variety of problems, including the prevention of child abuse and neglect and the parenting of children with special needs (Rickel & Becker, 1997). Provision of such support has been associated with positive outcomes, in general. Findings indicate the majority of parents (72 percent in a national study) cited emotional support as the most important aspect of this approach.

Ruch-Ross et al. (1992) compared 1004 OPF participants to 790 teen mothers (i.e., girls who gave birth at age 19 or younger) drawn from the database of the National Longitudinal Survey of Youth (NLSY) conducted by Ohio State University. Both groups were ethnically and racially diverse: the OPF group was 51.3 percent black, 41.8 percent white, and 6.9 percent Hispanic; the NLSY sample was 33 percent black, 46.8 percent White, and 19.4 percent Hispanic. OPF mothers tended to be younger than NLSY mothers, with the majority of NLSY mothers giving birth between ages 18 and 19, while most of the OPF mothers were under 18 when they gave birth.

Despite these differences in group composition, the NLSY mothers were 1.4 times more likely to have a second pregnancy during the 12-month follow-up period than were the OPF mothers, after investigators controlled for age at first birth, ethnic background, living arrangements, education, school enrollment, and employment at baseline (Ruch-Ross et al., 1992). In addition, the mothers who received the OPF intervention were 3.4 times more likely to be in school a year later, and 1.5 times more likely to be employed than the NLSY mothers, again after controlling for the differences in group composition. All of these findings were statistically significant (p < .05).

Once again, these findings suggest that providing interventions for teen mothers pays off in multiple ways, which have ramifications not only for the young women themselves and their children, but also for the larger society. If the United States is serious about reducing the welfare rolls, these studies suggest we would do well to provide sustained, well-planned, and supportive programs for teen mothers.

Recommendations from Researchers

Intervention technology has grown rapidly in the last two decades, spurred in part by the HIV epidemic. Although we are constantly learning more about what works in preventing and changing problem behaviors, funding for prevention and intervention has continued to diminish, with serious cuts in the 1990s to research and to direct services (Rickel & Becker, 1997).

Based on their review of 77 intervention studies, Choi and Coates (1994) provided several recommendations for the development of programs for prevention of HIV infection, which also have relevance for prevention of all types of high-risk sexual behavior:

1. Behavior changes that endure are more likely when interventions are continuous and repetitive over time.
2. Greater behavior change occurs the more intensive the intervention (i.e., multiple exposure over time leads to the greatest changes).
3. The accessibility of preventive measures is key to their effectiveness (e.g., condoms, clean needles).
4. Building behavioral skills and shifting community norms are important aspects of behavioral change.
5. Timing is a key variable in the success of programs, particularly with adolescents (e.g., interventions before youth become sexually active are more effective than later interventions).

6. Individual interventions are less powerful than those aimed at communities.
7. In high-risk groups, targeted interventions for couples where one partner is HIV positive may prevent the spread of the virus to the other partner.
8. HIV counseling and testing is important, but insufficient to reduce the risk of HIV transmission.
9. Community interventions, such as outreach and mobilization of resources, can be effective in modifying high-risk practices.
10. Media campaigns can be used to change behaviors of large populations.

The authors (Choi & Coates, 1994) noted dramatic gaps in the available literature for high-risk populations. Specifically, studies of women, younger gay and bisexual men, nonwhite gay or bisexual men, young adults not in college, adolescent drop-outs, patients with STDs, military personnel, and incarcerated groups were notably missing. Highest risk groups predicted for the 1990s (Coates, 1990) are (1) gay and bisexual men who live outside the areas hit hardest by the AIDS epidemic (e.g., San Francisco, New York); (2) ethnic minorities, particularly women and gay men; (3) clients of clinics for STDs and family planning; and (4) persons over 50 years of age. An important direction for future research will be interventions and evaluation studies directed at these key groups.

SUGGESTIONS FOR INTERVENTION

Based on the research and intervention work reviewed in this chapter, the following conclusions may be drawn.

Strategies Most Likely to Be Effective

Although education alone has been shown to be ineffective, a combination of increasing knowledge, increasing motivation, and enhancing competencies has a better chance of changing actual behavior. The educational aspects of any program are more likely to be effective when they are presented in culturally sensitive ways. Attention to cognitive developmental factors also increases the effectiveness of an intervention.

Assessing the stage of change of an individual or a group of individuals (e.g., college students) who are targeted for an intervention may enhance its effectiveness. Specifically, for individuals who are in the precontemplation stage about changing their risky sexual behavior, the advantages and benefits of changing unsafe practices should be strongly emphasized. However, for those in the contemplation stage, it may be more important to decrease their perceptions of the cost of making a change (such as hassles of using condoms or negative reaction of partners), in order to move them further into the action or maintenance phases of change. This is an important point in light of the finding that the best predictor of condom use was prior use, because those prior users, in the action stage by definition, may benefit from this de-emphasis of the disadvantages of using condoms, in order to keep them moving toward the maintenance stage with their behavior.

In conjunction with other strategies, raising individual perceptions of risk also appears to be an important and necessary component of change. The optimistic bias found in most populations is a cognitive factor that must be impacted for consciousness-raising to occur. Considerable evidence, as well as several theoretical models, suggests that the use of peer leaders is a powerful technique for changing perceptions of risk and for encouraging safe sex behavior. The teaching of "one-liners" that are easily used in sexual situations and help adolescents feel they are maintaining their "cool" may prove to be effective strategies for helping teens negotiate safer sex practices.

Use of videos showing individuals similar to the target group talking about and demonstrating strategies, or talking about how they contracted AIDS through mistakes made by most teens, provide effective means of communicating information in a way that adolescents can accept. The use of presenters who are similar to the audience or who are peer leaders, or "trendsetters," has been found to be effective across groups, including African-American women, gay men, and teens.

In general, interventions appear to be most effective before teens become sexually active, suggesting prevention education should begin early. Assessing individual personality factors may also be important in designing specific interventions, particularly in clinical settings where one-on-one interactions are used. Successful teen pregnancy

prevention strategies in clinic settings have stressed in-depth counseling, developmentally appropriate education, reassurance, and social
support. Interventions with teen mothers, aimed at delaying a second
pregnancy, were most successful when the teen participated for seven
weeks or more. Provision of a support structure for the teen during the
critical two months following birth appeared to have a significant
positive effect on her ability to make decisions which enhanced her
development and her child's future.

Finally, pregnant and parenting teens appear to be better off when
provided with a structured program of home visitation and parent
support groups. Again, such programs incorporate the key elements of
education, social support, and teaching of competencies common to all
effective interventions for reducing high-risk sexual behavior.

Strategies that Don't Work

Most individual elements are insufficient to produce the comprehensive changes necessary to reduce high-risk sexual behavior and
maintain safe sex practices. For example, education alone does not
change behavior, and neither does the teaching of negotiation skills
alone. Students report they often felt unable or ineffective in attempting
to use negotiation skills in complicated sexual situations, and knowledge of transmission of HIV or other STDs does not equal use of
protection against them. No program is likely to succeed that does not
incorporate multiple approaches to changing behavior.

4

Guidelines for Prevention, I
Ethnicity and Social Class
Considerations

Developing and implementing successful interventions often depend upon effectively addressing ethnicity and social class factors, as these influence sexual behavior and its risks. Sexual attitudes differ across cultures. In most cultures, there are strong standards regarding sexual behavior which differ for men and women. Cultural differences also affect the extent to which early sexual behavior is considered acceptable.

Poverty interacts with ethnicity in creating and maintaining risk factors. That is, the overrepresentation of some ethnic groups in poverty leads to increased risk for individual members of the group. Drug use and its association with increased sexual activity and the spread of HIV infection is also related to low socioeconomic status.

In this chapter, we examine cultural factors that influence sexual behavior, including how and to what extent such factors increase the risks for HIV and other STDs, as well as other negative consequences of sexual activity. We will also examine the implications for changing high-risk behaviors and, based on the research, offer guidelines regarding strategies that are likely to work, those that may be effective, and those that are unlikely to bring about behavior change for various ethnic populations.

CULTURAL ASPECTS OF RISK FOR
AFRICAN AMERICANS

African Americans are at higher risk for contracting HIV than are Caucasians. In 1992, although African Americans accounted for 12 percent of the U.S. population, they made up 29 percent of AIDS cases that year (Centers for Disease Control, 1992). Lack of knowledge about HIV may be a reason for higher levels of risk for minorities. In a nationwide survey of more than 71,000 subjects, Sweat and Levin (1995) examined differences in knowledge about HIV in relation to ethnicity and socioeconomic status (SES). They found that ethnic minority subjects and those from lower SES groups knew fewer facts about HIV, including ways that HIV is transmitted. However, they also found SES to be more predictive of HIV knowledge than was ethnicity.

Minority women are at great risk for contracting HIV through heterosexual contact. African American and Hispanic women are 11 times more likely than white women to become infected with the AIDS virus through heterosexual transmission (Holmes, Karon, & Kreiss, 1990). Such risks to women may be due in part to prevailing attitudes in the culture regarding sexual behavior. African Americans reportedly have fewer biases against early sexual activity among adolescents (Marsiglio, 1989), an acceptance which, in past decades, may have resulted in higher rates of pregnancy among unmarried African-American adolescents than among their white counterparts. Today, however, the spread of HIV has also become a pressing health issue for the African-American community.

Marsiglio (1989) summarizes theories that may explain these patterns of earlier sexual behavior among African Americans. Of primary relevance to the expectations regarding family structure and child rearing is the bleak economic situation faced by many African Americans. African-American men may be less likely to be considered as potential means of support for women and their children, making the institution of marriage less desirable. Also, within the African-American community, early sexual activity and pregnancy before marriage are more acceptable than in the population at large.

Likewise, higher rates of incarceration among young African-American males limit the opportunities for many African-American women to form long-term partnerships with men of their own race (Weeks, Schensul, Williams, Singer, & Grier, 1995). As a result of this perceived scarcity, women might be less likely to insist on condom use or other safe sex practices that might be unacceptable to their partners. Contradicting that assertion, however, are the findings by Osmond and colleagues (1993) that African-American women were more effective than women of other ethnicities in convincing partners to use condoms. They attribute this difference in part to the fact that African-American women in their study were less reliant on their partners for financial support and, therefore, had more power in their relationships.

Crack use is also a risk factor for increased sexual behavior among African-American youth (Bowser et al., 1990). Poverty too often denies young people living in inner cities opportunities, so that they may be easily lured into drug use, drug dealing, and the consequences of these activities. Delaying sexual activity for the uncertain goal of becoming educated and financially better off is rarely seen as a viable option for African-American youth from economically depressed neighborhoods, whereas drug dealing may bring immediate financial gains. Using crack and other drugs is associated with higher frequencies of sexual activity, as well as higher numbers of risky sexual behaviors. Therefore, drug users as well as sexual partners of drug users are placed at higher risk for contracting HIV and other STDs.

Because risks to African-American youth abound in the environment, the chances of contracting HIV may not seem a viable threat to those most at risk. Stevenson and Davis (1994) point out that the very real possibility of being murdered poses a more apparent risk to African-American teenagers than does becoming infected with a disease that will end their lives as much as a decade or more in the future (see Table 4.1).

Barriers to Change for African Americans

For African Americans, economics is a major factor that promotes and maintains high-risk sexual behavior (Bowser et al., 1990). African-American youth often see their chances for a prosperous and satisfying adulthood as limited, and in many cases may not expect to survive the threat of violent crime present daily in their neighborhoods (Stevenson & Davis, 1994).

Table **4.1**. Ten Leading Causes of Death for Black and White Youth,
Compared to the Total U.S. Population[a]

U.S. population, all groups	Blacks, age 15 to 24		Whites, age 15 to 24	
	Males	Females	Males	Females
1. Heart disease	Homicide	Homicide	Accidents	Accidents
2. Cancer	Accidents	Accidents	Suicide	Homicide
3. Stroke	Suicide	HIV/AIDS	Homicide	Suicide
4. Chronic obstructive pulmonary disease (COPD)	Heart disease	Heart disease	Malignancies	Malignancies
5. Accidents	HIV/AIDS	Malignancies	Heart disease	Heart disease
6. Pneumonia/influenza	Malignancies	Suicide	Congenital anomalies	Congenital anomalies
7. Diabetes	COPD	Anemias	HIV/AIDS	HIV/AIDS
8. HIV/AIDS	Anemias	Pregnancy/ childbirth	Pneumonia/ influenza	COPD
9. Suicide	Congenital anomalies	COPD	Cerebrovascular diseases	Pneumonia/ influenza
10. Chronic liver disease/ cirrhosis	Diabetes	Congenital anomalies	COPD	Cerebrovascular diseases

[a]Source: Anderson, R. N., Kochanek, K. D., & Murphy, S. L. (1997). Report of final mortality statistics, 1995. *Monthly Vital Statistics Report*, 45 (11, Supplement 2), National Center for Health Statistics.

Drug use and involvement with the selling of drugs, particularly crack cocaine, are interwoven with the economic plight and the risky sexual behavior that are ravaging the African-American community (Bowser et al., 1990). Because crack use and the selling of crack often take place in exchange for sex, and because African-American youth are at particularly high risk for being drawn into the business of drugs, the risk of contracting HIV cannot be separated from using and dealing in crack. Likewise, the existence and preponderance of crack use and sales go hand-in-hand with the economic plight of inner-city African Americans who have been systematically excluded from mainstream economic opportunities.

Without the prospect of completing an education or finding a good job that motivates those with a greater number of options (including higher-status black youth), disadvantaged African-American youth have little reason to postpone sexual activity. Bowser et al. (1990) summarize the effect of early sexual activity for these youth: "The social meaning of early teen sexuality is that these young people have opted out of long-term adolescence because of a lack of economic mobility" (p. 60).

In a survey of 222 crack users in 1988 (Bowser et al., 1990), 42 percent reported at least one incidence of being diagnosed with an STD. The highest rates of infection were found among those who both sold crack and used drugs in association with sexual activity. Fifty-nine percent of adolescent crack users reported having used a condom at least once, but only 20 percent reported using a condom the last time they had sex. While the sale of crack, and the sexual activity that takes place in exchange for it, often occurs within the setting of crack houses, prostitution and other risky behaviors are related to the use of crack as well.

Another barrier to prevention for the African-American community is the often justified mistrust of white society and its intentions (Stevenson & Davis 1994). Efforts to promote the use of birth control in African-American communities have traditionally been seen as an effort by whites to reduce the African-American population. Since condoms have traditionally been used primarily as a means of birth control, there may be some expectation among African Americans that programs designed to increase condom use are really efforts to limit the African-American population, and some African Americans may even see the AIDS virus as a white-initiated strategy for reducing the number of African Americans in the United States (Stevenson & White, 1990).

St. Lawrence (1993) enumerates reasons that African-American adolescents may be reluctant to use condoms. Among these are the belief that condoms decrease sensation during intercourse and the inconvenience of using condoms. Also, the use of drugs and alcohol may cloud judgment, reducing one's resolve to practice safe sex.

Perhaps the most interesting and challenging objection to using condoms by African-American adolescents cited by St. Lawrence (1993) is the misconception of members of many high-risk groups that their risk is relatively low. This author suggests that African Americans may not recognize the risks they face because most interventions and educational campaigns focusing on HIV infection have targeted white gay men. Weeks and colleagues (1995) make the point that prevention programs have recently focused on middle-class populations, including transmission by heterosexual contact and transmission to children. Yet some of the highest risk groups, such as minority adolescents, have not always been adequately addressed in prevention efforts.

CULTURAL ASPECTS OF RISK
TO HISPANICS

The Centers for Disease Control (1996b) report that while the AIDS epidemic has begun to stabilize for the white population, the spread of AIDS continues to grow for Hispanics and African Americans. For Hispanic men, 37 percent of AIDS cases are contracted through injection drug use, compared to 25 percent of AIDS cases resulting from injection drug use for the population at large. For Hispanic women, injection drug use accounts for 44 percent of AIDS cases. Heterosexual contact is responsible for 45 percent of AIDS cases for Hispanic females, while for white women 35 percent of cases are attributed to heterosexual contact.

Heterosexual transmission of AIDS is growing at a faster rate for Hispanics than for any other ethnic group in the United States (Centers for Disease Control, 1994a). From 1992 to 1993, the rate of heterosexually transmitted AIDS increased 126 percent for Hispanic males and 147 percent for Hispanic females, as compared to 106 percent for white males and 145 percent for white females, and 112 percent for African-American males and 131 percent for African-American females. In 1993, Hispanic males accounted for 23 percent of males with heterosexually transmitted AIDS. In the same year, Hispanic women made up 24 percent of females with AIDS acquired through heterosexual activity. Hispanics are also at high risk for AIDS transmission related to injection drug use (Centers for Disease Control, 1996a). From July 1994 to June 1995, the Centers for Disease Control estimated that rates of opportunistic illnesses associated with AIDS for Hispanics were eight times those of whites (Centers for Disease Control, 1995).

In general, Hispanic populations in the United States are concentrated in areas with high prevalence rates of HIV infection (Marin & Gomez, 1997). However, for those who live in the Northeast (who are primarily from Puerto Rico and the Dominican Republic), the risk of HIV infection is greater than for those residing in the Southwest (who primarily come from Mexico and Central and South America) (Selik, Castro, & Pappaioanou, 1988). This difference is believed to be related to higher rates of injection drug use, greater numbers of sexual partners, and more sexual activity between men (Marin & Gomez, 1997). The rates of reported cases in the Southwest may be lower because of immigration laws which prohibit HIV-infected persons from immigrating to the United States. Reluctance on the part of undocumented workers to seek public services may also decrease the numbers of reported cases in the Southwest.

Cultural Differences regarding Attitudes about Sex

Prevailing attitudes about sex and sex roles within a culture determine the kinds and frequency of sexual behaviors in which individuals engage. In the Hispanic population, sex roles often remain very traditional, particularly for those who are less acculturated (Marin & Gomez, 1997). Women are under a great deal of pressure not to engage in sex before marriage or outside of marriage. For Hispanic men, however, there is less pressure to refrain from sex outside of marriage, or even to practice monogamy within marriage.

Marin, Gomez, and Hearst (1993) conducted a telephone survey sampling Hispanics in the Northeast and Southwest. In their survey, 60 percent of unmarried men reported having multiple sex partners in the previous 12-month period. Likewise, 18 percent of married Hispanic men reported having multiple partners, compared to 9 percent of married non-Hispanic white men. In contrast, only 15 percent of unmarried and 3 percent of married Hispanic women reported having multiple partners.

In a study by Van Oss-Marin, Tschann, Gomez, and Kegeles (1993), Spanish-speaking Hispanic women had fewer sexual partners and were less likely to use condoms than white women. Furthermore, these Hispanic women had negative attitudes about condom use and expressed less confidence in their ability to avoid contracting HIV.

According to Osmond and colleagues (1993), Hispanic women living in the United States are being exposed to a more sexually liberal environment, but are still bound to traditional views about sex and birth control. In particular, these women's choices are influenced by the doctrines of the Catholic church, which forbid the use of contraception, including condoms.

Yet another issue is that Hispanic women are taught to behave submissively toward men (Osmond et al., 1993). According to Marin and Gomez (1997), very different standards exist in the Hispanic culture regarding what is considered acceptable behavior in sexual matters for men and women. In most Hispanic cultures, women are expected to be virgins at the time that they marry. Those who are not virgins at marriage are considered immoral, so that women are under a great deal of pressure to refrain from sex. Hispanic men who are interested in having sex may be reluctant to talk to potential sex partners about condom use or sex in general. Hispanic men report they believe that their partners are often ambivalent about having sex from the outset, and that taking the time to discuss condoms or obtain condoms might result in their partners changing their minds and refusing to have sex at all.

Hispanic women are also taught to avoid open communication about sex (Osmond et al., 1993). Some studies have found that a common belief of Hispanics is that moral women should not know about sex. In a study by Marin and Gomez (1997), 25 percent of their subjects said that it is disrespectful for men to talk to women about sex, and 20 percent said that it was "dangerous" (p. 79) for women to be as knowledgeable about sex as a man.

Osmond et al. (1993) also note that negative attitudes toward homosexuality might induce bisexual men to marry, thus increasing the spread of HIV through heterosexual activity. Marin and Gomez (1997) found that only about 20 percent of their sample approved of sexual relations between men and approximately two-thirds of the sample found homosexuality "distasteful" (p. 80).

Although many traditional attitudes may prevail in the culture at large, Hispanic adolescents in the United States become sexually active earlier than other adolescents. As a result, they show higher rates of teen pregnancy and of infection with HIV and other STDs (Marin & Gomez, 1997). In one study conducted in a school in California, 24 percent of Hispanic adolescents in the sixth through eighth grades reported having had sex, as compared to 18 percent of all subjects in the sample.

Such rates of early sexual activity are particularly disturbing considering that Hispanic parents may be reluctant to talk to their children about sex. Marin and Gomez (1997) suggest that children receive very little, if any, information from their parents about sex. Usually the information that is given tends to be vague or sketchy, such as a warning to "be careful," without elaboration on how or why (p. 81).

Hispanics may also be experiencing higher rates of sexual coercion. Marin and Gomez (1997) found that 73 percent of a sample of sexually active Hispanic women reported being pressured during the last year to have sex when they would have preferred not to do so. Ninety-two percent of the men in the sample reported pressuring a partner when she did not want to have sex. The study's authors attribute such tendencies to the lack of equality in relationships, and to the perception that men are unable to control their passion.

Barriers to Change for Hispanics

Clearly the inequality between the sexes is a significant obstacle to fighting the spread of HIV in the Hispanic community (Marin & Gomez, 1997). As long as it is unacceptable for women to acquire knowledge about sex, much less to be assertive about sexual matters, men will hold the greater share of power in determining sexual practices, both for themselves and for their wives or partners. To complicate matters, since married and unmarried Hispanic men report having multiple sex partners at a much higher rate than do Hispanic women, even women who believe they are involved in monogamous relationships may be in danger of contracting HIV. At the same time, women are more likely than men to contract HIV through heterosexual intercourse, placing them in a very risky situation.

However, despite these factors, many Hispanics report always using condoms with secondary sex partners (Marin & Gomez, 1997). Hispanics also report using condoms to about the same extent as others do. Interestingly, 56 percent of Hispanic men and women in a recent survey reported that, when they were younger, an older person talked to them about condoms and endorsed their use.

Less acculturated Hispanic men were found to be far more likely to carry condoms (Marin, Tschann, Gomez, & Kegeles, 1993). In one sample, 82 percent of unmarried Hispanic men and women who carried condoms used them, whereas only 27 percent of those who did not carry condoms reported using condoms during their most recent sexual experience (Marin, Gomez, & Tschann, 1993). For Hispanics, a major issue for condom use appears to be the availability of prophylactics (as it is for many other groups).

Purchasing condoms may be a major obstacle for many Hispanics. Marin and Gomez (1997) explain that condoms are frequently reported to be shoplifted by Hispanics because they are too embarrassed to buy them or because of their cost. Making condoms available, affordable, and accessible, and minimizing the embarrassment associated with their purchase, may be a key component of an HIV-prevention program in the Hispanic community.

Another potential risk factor for the Hispanic community is the recently discovered high rate of anal sex among this population. In a study of men age 20 to 39 (Billy, Tanfer, Grady, & Klepinger, 1993), 23 percent of Hispanics reported having had anal sex in the past four months, compared to 21 percent of African Americans, and 9 percent of non-Hispanic whites. Anal sex is the most high-risk sexual act. The rectum's vulnerability to tissue damage during intercourse, compared to the vagina (e.g., breaks in the tissue are more likely to occur during anal than during vaginal sex), allows HIV transmission from seminal fluid into the bloodstream of the receptive partner (Kalichman, 1995).

Anal intercourse is sometimes seen as an alternative to vaginal intercourse in order to prevent pregnancy. Gayle and D'Angelo (1991) found that one-quarter of the adolescent girls in their study reported engaging in anal sex because of the absence of pregnancy risk, and because they saw this activity as one that did not compromise their virginity. Where this is the case, and when condoms are seen only as a contraceptive device, some couples who practice anal sex may not use condoms at all (Marin & Gomez, 1997).

RISKS TO ASIAN AMERICANS

Although Asian Americans still account for a small percentage overall of AIDS cases reported in the United States, their risk for contracting HIV is growing (Centers for Disease Control, 1994a). The Centers for Disease Control reported that for Asian and Pacific Islander males living in the United States, the number of reported AIDS cases caused by heterosexual contact increased from 3 to 16 from 1992 to 1993. For women of the same population, the corresponding increase was from 20 to 52 cases. So, while the actual number of cases is quite low, they are multiplying rapidly. Gay Asian and Pacific Islander men also face great risk, as 72 percent of AIDS cases reported for Asians are contracted through homosexual or bisexual activity (Centers for Disease Control, 1994b).

Barriers to Change for Asian Americans

Cultural factors may pose a challenge to intervention efforts for Asian Americans. Brown (1992) argues that Asian and Pacific Island cultures are collectivist in nature, while American culture tends to be more individualistic. Collectivist cultures emphasize the importance of groups and conceptualize values and activities in relation to ingroups and outgroups. For this reason, and because AIDS has typically been associated with homosexual activity, Brown believes that most members of such a culture would interpret AIDS as an outgroup phenomenon and, therefore, less of a personal threat.

Brown (1992) also describes differences in communication styles that might impact Asian Americans' behaviors related to safe sex. Talking about sex is not typically acceptable in most Asian cultures. In fact, Brown describes communication in general as being less direct and less self-disclosing. For these reasons, he concludes that communication about HIV is likely to be especially problematic for this population.

In a study at a university in the western United States, Brown (1992) tested two hypotheses: (1) Subjects with an Asian-Pacific cultural background would express less concern related to HIV than those with North American cultural backgrounds; and (2) those with Asian-Pacific cultural backgrounds would report lower levels of communication regarding HIV than those from North American backgrounds. His sample included 257 students, 69.6 percent of whom were of Asian-Pacific backgrounds. Fifty-one percent of the sample were female and 92.2 percent spoke English as their first language.

Both hypotheses were confirmed. In addition, Brown (1992) found that women of both cultural backgrounds reported higher levels of communication about HIV than men of either background. Also, North American women reported more concern regarding HIV than men of the same background, but for Asian-Pacific subjects, there was no significant difference between men and women related to degree of concern.

Brown (1992) suggests that because there seem to be cultural differences at work in Asian Americans' perception of AIDS, interventions should be designed to address these differences. For example, he recommends emphasizing that HIV can be spread through heterosexual activity and depicting Asian Americans in education and prevention materials. He also suggests using the collectivist nature of Asian-American culture to introduce AIDS education and communication through preexisting groups within the community.

In a study of HIV risk among Asian and Pacific Island gay men living in the San Francisco area, Choi and colleagues (Choi, Coates, Catania, Lew, & Chow, 1995) found that the occurrence of unprotected sex for Asian gay men in their study was higher than previously reported levels for white gay men. The Asian gay men in this study demonstrated high levels of knowledge about HIV, but only 17 percent expressed the belief that they were personally at risk for contracting HIV.

However, Choi et al. (1995) found that 59 percent of the Asian gay men in their study reported having multiple partners during the last three months, while 95 percent reported having multiple partners over the last five years. Thirteen percent of those who had been tested for HIV (78 percent of the sample) reported being HIV positive. Of those who were currently in a relationship, 13 percent reported having a primary partner who was HIV positive. The use of drugs and alcohol was found to be related to having unprotected anal sex.

Choi et al. (1995) emphasize the need to raise the awareness of Asian and Pacific Island gay men that they are at risk for AIDS. They suggest having Asians appear in media campaigns for HIV prevention, encouraging communication about HIV among sexual partners, and designing interventions to increase Asian gay men's levels of acceptance of themselves and their sexuality.

RISKS TO NATIVE AMERICANS

Native Americans and Alaskan Natives have relatively low rates of HIV infection compared to other ethnic groups (Centers for Disease

Control, 1994a). However, their rates of infection due to heterosexual contact are increasing. From 1992 to 1993, for males of these ethnic groups, the number of AIDS cases related to heterosexual activity rose from 1 to 6, while the rates for females rose from 5 to 23 cases.

Warren et al. (1990) studied sexual behavior of Native Americans in Montana. Subjects were members of the Blackfeet tribe, and included individuals living on a reservation and those living in the city of Great Falls. These authors report that Native Americans in their sample were more likely than whites to have had intercourse before the age of 17. Subjects living on the reservation reported higher rates of contraceptive use than those living in Great Falls (79 percent and 58 percent, respectively). However, condoms were not a popular form of contraception. For female respondents on the reservation and in town, 4.2 percent reported using condoms, compared to 4.0 percent of African-American women and 9.8 percent of white women in the United States. The most frequently used methods were female sterilization, birth-control pills, and IUDs.

Warren et al. (1990) also examined substance use during pregnancy among this population. Of the subjects living in Great Falls, approximately 60 percent reported smoking cigarettes and 36 percent reported drinking alcohol during their most recent pregnancy. Those living on the reservation reported somewhat more conservative behavior in this respect, with 33 percent and 14 percent reporting tobacco and alcohol use, respectively, during their last pregnancies. The rates for smoking during pregnancy for white and African-American women in the United States is 28 percent, while rates for alcohol consumption during pregnancy for African Americans are comparable to those of Native Americans living in Great Falls. According to Warren et al. (1990), white women report higher rates of drinking during pregnancy than any other group.

Conner and Conner (1992) examined Native-American adolescents' attitudes about alcohol use. They note that alcohol use is higher for young Native Americans than for youth of other groups. These authors were interested in beliefs about alcohol that might encourage high-risk sexual behavior. They refer to a 1990 report of the Indian Health Service that stressed that Native Americans are at risk for heterosexually transmitted HIV because of high rates of pregnancy and use of alcohol.

The authors (Conner & Conner, 1992) were interested in examining the beliefs that motivate Native-American youth to combine alcohol with sexual behavior. They hypothesized that alcohol use related to sexual activity might be related to two different conceptualizations about the benefits of alcohol: (1) Alcohol might be seen as a means of reducing anxiety around sexual activity, or (2) alcohol might be believed to heighten enjoyment of the sexual experience. Conner and Conner argue that the latter belief might be associated with heavier drinking and would be likely to lead to higher rates of risky sexual behavior.

To answer these questions, Conner and Conner (1992) surveyed 42 Native-American adolescents (21 males and 21 females) ranging in age from 14 to 17 years. These young people were from different tribes and five different states and had come together at a powwow, where the study was conducted.

Sixty percent of the subjects reported that they had not used alcohol during the powwow, while 40 percent had. Sixty-eight percent of the subjects endorsed one or more items on a teen behavior survey indicating they believed drinking alcohol increases sexual pleasure. Seventy-four percent expressed the belief that alcohol reduces the anxiety associated with sexual situations. Male subjects were more likely to report drinking heavily. Heavier drinking was correlated with the expectation that drinking increases sexual pleasure.

Conner and Conner (1992) emphasize the danger inherent in these behaviors and attitudes in relation to the potential for the spread of HIV among Native Americans. Suggesting further research to clarify the reasons behind these demonstrated expectations, the authors question whether these beliefs may be explained by lack of knowledge about drinking, by some relationship to childhood abuse, or may be attributable to some other as yet unknown cause.

Even though the rates of HIV infection are increasing for Native Americans, little research has been done regarding their risk for HIV and the efficacy of prevention strategies with this population. Considering the low frequency of condom usage reported by Warren et al. (1990) and the relatively early age of first intercourse reported in the same study, this population should be studied further and targeted for HIV-prevention strategies.

INTERVENTIONS FOR ETHNIC MINORITIES

Many of the barriers to prevention of high-risk sexual behavior and the spread of HIV for members of ethnic minorities are related to poverty and the social problems it creates. Therefore, changing the political and economic forces that perpetuate the current conditions will be necessary to achieve lasting changes for those who face the greatest risks. Poverty, the drug trade, and high-risk sexual behavior are interrelated and serve to maintain the limited prospects that face inner-city youth, as Bowser and colleagues (1990) point out.

Meanwhile, prevention efforts should focus on helping members of ethnic minorities recognize the risks they face and provide them with usable strategies to prevent the spread of HIV. In this section, we will examine some of the research regarding the types of interventions that are likely to be most effective with ethnic minorities. Most of these interventions involve some form of education promoting competence regarding safe sex practices. Specifically many of these educational interventions include information about risky sexual behaviors, the transmission of HIV, and how to prevent becoming infected. Other factors that will be examined include the effects of culturally tailored interventions, integrating the values and social context of the ethnic community into the message, and challenging cultural beliefs that may be detrimental.

Fisher and Fisher (1992) devised the IMB model for behavior change related to HIV risk. This model emphasizes that for high-risk sexual behavior to be reduced, the target audience must receive information about HIV risk, must be motivated to change their be-havior, and must be taught specific behavioral skills that will result in decreased risk. Fisher and Fisher argue that only when all three of these conditions are met will behavior change actually take place. This model has been supported by research with various populations (Fisher et al., 1994). While most of the interventions described in this chapter include some or all of these components, it seems likely that those which use the full IMB model would produce the most powerful outcomes. See Chapter 3 for a more complete discussion of this model.

Strategies for Prevention Programs for African Americans

Considering the barriers to change in the African-American community, Bowser and colleagues (1990) suggest that an effective strategy for reducing the risk of HIV to African Americans should incorporate several key elements. First, because high-risk sexual behavior and the risk of HIV infection are so integrally tied to the state of the economy in African-American communities, the first step is to improve the economic conditions faced by inner-city African Americans. These communities will have to be revitalized and brought into the mainstream of the American economy, offering their youth the possibility of a decent life, the promise of which will provide motivation to refrain from early and risky sexual behaviors and involvement with drugs and other illegal activities.

Interventions aimed at inner-city African Americans will have to be based in or near the public housing projects where drug sales take place and should be headed by members of the community itself (Bowser et al., 1990). The function of those external to the community should be to provide support for those implementing the programs. Stopping the drug trade in these areas is essential, yet ending the drug traffic will depend upon preventing the sale of drugs to those outside the community. For example, in San Francisco and Oakland, most of the sale of crack takes place within the public housing projects. However, in those cities, most of the income from crack sales within the projects comes from customers who drive into the neighborhood to purchase crack. Therefore, eliminating crack trafficking from these neighborhoods will require wiping out this exploitation of inner-city neighborhoods by drug dealers and purchasers from outside the area.

Research on Interventions Aimed at Minority Populations

In this section, we examine empirical studies that have tested the outcomes of various types of interventions with different at-risk minority populations. The studies examine the efficacy of strategies such as neighborhood-based interventions, matching the ethnicity of the individuals implementing the intervention to the target audience, and matching gender of the target audience to gender of those who present the information or are teaching the skills.

One such study (Jemmott, Jemmott, & Fong, 1992) was designed to reduce the frequency of risky sexual behaviors leading to HIV and other sexually transmitted diseases in male African-American adolescents. The intervention was based in Philadelphia and included 157 adolescents recruited from a medical clinic, local high schools, and a YMCA. The mean age of subjects was 14.64 years; 97 percent were in school.

The intervention lasted five hours and consisted of videos, games, and other activities. The materials were designed to be culturally consistent with the audience and to be engaging to the age group. The intervention provided educational information about AIDS, a "basketball" game that involved correctly answering questions about AIDS, and an exercise in which participants engaged in role-playing the negotiation of safe sex practices.

A comparison group spent the same amount of time in a similarly designed set of activities that focused, instead of on AIDS prevention, on career choices. Jemmott et al. (1992) used the control situation to avoid any effects that might be attributed to the AIDS intervention solely because the adolescent boys were involved in a group activity in which they received attention from adults.

After the intervention, participants in the AIDS prevention group reported fewer intentions to participate in high-risk sexual behaviors, more negative attitudes toward high-risk sexual behaviors, and higher levels of knowledge about AIDS than did those subjects in the control career condition. Subjects in the AIDS group who had a male facilitator reported higher levels of knowledge about AIDS than did those who had a female facilitator.

At the three-month follow-up, those from the AIDS prevention condition reported still having fewer intentions to participate in high-risk sexual acts than did those from the control group. Also during this three-month follow-up, the higher levels of knowledge about AIDS observed immediately postintervention were maintained.

Several interesting trends emerged with regard to the gender of facilitators who led the AIDS prevention groups (Jemmott et al., 1992). Negative attitudes about risky sexual behavior observed postintervention were maintained more effectively during the three-month follow-up by subjects in the group led by a female facilitator. Those subjects in the AIDS group with a male facilitator reported higher levels of knowledge about AIDS than did those with a female facilitator; however, after three months, the gender/knowledge effect had disappeared. At this follow-up point, subjects who had female facilitators reported engaging in fewer high-risk behaviors and maintaining more negative attitudes toward high-risk behaviors than did those who had male facilitators.

From these results, it is evident interventions aimed at young people can have lasting effects on their behavior and attitudes about risky sexual behavior. However, these results also suggest that, for male adolescents, matching the facilitator of an intervention to the gender of subjects is not particularly necessary nor more effective.

Some critics maintain that providing young people with information about AIDS or giving them condoms will entice adolescents into earlier and more frequent sexual activity. Sellers, McGraw, and McKinlay (1994) tested this hypothesis by creating an intervention for Hispanic youth in Boston. Their sample included 586 Hispanics between the ages of 14 and 20, but the intervention was designed to reach the specific neighborhoods in the community.

For this intervention, a comprehensive campaign was launched, designed to saturate the Hispanic adolescent population of chosen neighborhoods (Sellers et al., 1994). Their strategies included workshops conducted in schools, community organizations, and health centers. They held group discussions in the homes of Hispanic youth, ran television and radio ads, and put up posters in businesses and transit areas. They distributed kits door-to-door containing condoms and instructions on their use. They maintained an office where they distributed condoms without charge. The authors used Hartford, Connecticut, as a comparison city.

Two major benefits resulted from the intervention. First, males living in Boston were less likely to have become sexually active during the intervention than males living in Hartford. No such effect was observed for female subjects. Second, females in the study reduced the number of sex partners over the course of the intervention. No such effect was found for males. There was no effect on the frequency of sexual activity.

Because the intervention was aimed at the neighborhoods as a whole and not specifically at the 586 subjects whose behavior was evaluated before and after the intervention, not all of the subjects were actually exposed to the campaign. Therefore, the authors stress that the reported results are a somewhat conservative representation of the efficacy of the intervention.

Weeks et al. (1995) conducted an intervention called Project COPE (Community Outreach Prevention Effort), which was designed to bring AIDS education, counseling, and social services to injection drug users and sex partners of injection drug users. They recruited a sample of 934 subjects, composed of 714 men and 220 women. Of the total number of subjects, 734 were injection drug users (139 of whom were women) and 200 were sex partners of injection drug users (83 of whom were women). The women in the sample included 83 African Americans, 102 Hispanics, and 34 whites.

African Americans and Hispanics were assigned either to interventions that incorporated cultural values, presented by staff of the same ethnicity, or to a generic intervention along with the white subjects. The generic intervention included the same AIDS educational content, but did not address issues related to culture. For Hispanics in the culturally tailored intervention, values related to family and relationships were emphasized. Hispanic women were recruited by a Hispanic outreach worker and were seen in their homes, usually with family members and possibly with their sexual partners. African-American women received the intervention in groups and were not seen in their homes. For African-American women, the concepts of pride and religion were integrated into the intervention.

The ethnically matched interventions also included information about social issues, including racism and social class differences, relevant to the spread of AIDS. The authors report that these topics were discussed in ways designed to empower the women to find solutions or methods for dealing effectively with these problems.

Women who participated in the ethnically targeted interventions were found to be more likely to complete the program than those in the generic condition (Weeks et al., 1995). This result held both for Hispanic and African-American women. The researchers also found that more injection drug users than sex partners of drug users remained in the program until its completion. The authors suggested the latter finding may mean that sex partners of drug users felt the program was targeted less for them and more toward the drug users themselves. They also speculated that attrition for African-American women would have been lower had their interventions taken place in same-sex groups.

This study indicates that culturally sensitive interventions may hold participants' interest longer than programs designed for more generic audiences. Interventions in the home that include family members and sex partners also may be more effective for some groups. Gender differences may be a barrier to participation when mixed gender groups consist of individuals who did not previously know one another.

SUGGESTIONS FOR INTERVENTIONS

Further research is needed to properly address the question of how best to design interventions for various ethnic groups. Furthermore, while this is true of ethnic minorities in general, research regarding interventions with Asian Americans and Native Americans is particularly scarce.

Successful Interventions

Considering the outcomes of the studies outlined in this chapter, interventions that address the following issues seem to be most effective. Interventions based on the IMB model should be highly successful. These programs will provide education about risks, increase the motivation of the target audience to reduce risky behaviors, and will provide training in behaviors that will result in safer sex practices.

Interventions should also be designed based on cultural aspects of the targeted ethnic group. Programs for Hispanics should emphasize family and community and should be consistent with supporting these values. Interventions for African Americans should focus on the practice of safe sex as a factor of one's pride and in keeping with religious beliefs. Asian Americans are likely to be best served by programs that are introduced into preexisting groups within the culture and which can be integrated into a collectivist model, rather than strategies that would require the target audience to take action in a more individualistic way.

Successful interventions should be tailored to the gender of the potential audience. In intervening with women, cultural beliefs that limit women's willingness to challenge the authority of men in sexual situations must be addressed. Interventions for Hispanic women were more successful when conducted in their homes with family members and sexual partners present.

Interventions should be planned and executed by members of the ethnic groups and communities that they address. Financial and organizational support should be provided as needed, but control should be maintained by those within the community.

Condoms should be made readily available. They should be inexpensive and sold from vending machines or through other means that allow them to be purchased anonymously. Because condoms are a reasonably effective means of prevention of HIV and other STDs, media campaigns should be used to improve attitudes about their use.

Strategies that May Succeed

While education alone is insufficient to produce behavior change, research shows that members of most ethnic minorities may lack basic knowledge of HIV and the degree to which they are at risk. Interventions should be designed that specifically target these groups and prevention materials should include models or spokespersons who are members of the target ethnicity.

For Native Americans, there have been very few attempts at understanding or reducing the risk of unsafe sex. For this population, educational programs should be designed to increase the use of condoms for the prevention of STDs and pregnancy and to raise awareness about the effects of alcohol and its effect on high-risk sexual behavior.

Unsuccessful Strategies

Generically designed programs that stress HIV education but do not address cultural issues have been less successful than culturally sensitive interventions. Interventions presented to groups of mixed gender individuals may lead to attrition among group members, and may therefore fail to produce the desired results.

Interventions that target minorities whose risky behaviors are affected by poverty and associated problems are not likely to be successful until social programs can be put in place to address these societal issues. AIDS and teen pregnancy prevention cannot be properly addressed without attention to the social problems that increase these threats to ethnic minorities. Community efforts must address poverty issues, such as bringing economic and educational opportunities to the youth of inner cities. Only then will the drug addiction and trafficking that exacerbate the problems of risky sexual behavior be eliminated.

5

Guidelines for Intervention, II
Women

Women are particularly at risk for negative consequences of sexual behavior. Traditionally, women have been subject to the larger share of responsibility for preventing pregnancy and for dealing with outcomes of unplanned pregnancies. With the risks of contracting HIV and other STDs on the rise, the stakes associated with unprotected sex become much higher. These risks are compounded for women living in poverty. Table 5.1 shows ethnic differences in reported cases of AIDS for U.S. women in 1996.

Specific factors and consequences for women are outlined in this chapter. Issues discussed here include the ways in which women may feel compelled to engage in sexual behaviors due to intimidation, coercion, or violence in intimate relationships; how sexual assault poses threats to a woman's ability to exercise choice over her own behavior; and how a history of childhood sexual abuse may be associated with exploitation and revictimization in adulthood. Poverty increases the risk for women, with poor women most at risk for negative outcomes of sexual behavior.

In this chapter, women's use of alcohol and other drugs and its association with risky sexual activity are discussed. Use of substances lessens inhibition and leads to increased risk-taking. The use of alcohol and other drugs during pregnancy can have detrimental effects on infants. Women whose sexual partners are injection drug users are highly vulnerable to HIV infection.

Table 5.1. AIDS Cases in Women by Race/Ethnicity,
per 100,000 Women, Reported in 1996[a]

Race/ethnicity	Numbers	Percentage of cases
Black, non-Hispanic	8,147	59
White, non-Hispanic	2,888	21
Hispanic	2,629	19
Asian/Pacific Islander	81	1
American Indian/Alaska native	41	<1
Ethnicity unknown	34	<1
Totals	13,820	100

[a]Source: Centers for Disease Control and Prevention, HIV/AIDS Prevention Program (1997, September). www.cdc.gov/nchstp/hiv_aids/graphics/women.htm

HIV can be transmitted to fetuses by HIV-positive mothers. Children born with AIDS have extensive and progressive medical problems, as well as very short life expectancies. These issues will be explored further in this chapter. Finally, strategies for intervention with women are presented which target increased condom use, changing women's perceptions of risk in sexual activity, and enhancing women's assertiveness in sexual relationships.

In this chapter we will discuss various strategies for intervention with women. We will end the chapter by suggesting guidelines for interventions based on the research reviewed. We will discuss strategies that have been shown to be successful, those that may be effective, and strategies that are not likely to work.

PARTNER INTIMIDATION, COERCION, AND VIOLENCE

Women find themselves in sexual relationships for a variety of reasons other than their own clear preferences. Many women report that they engaged in their earliest sexual experiences out of curiosity or because of peer pressure (Wyatt & Riederle, 1994). Often, women remain in unsatisfying relationships with men because of economic pressures, concerns about the welfare of their children, or the threat of violence should they attempt to leave the relationship. They may fear retaliation if they refuse their partner's request for sexual intercourse.

Because of differences in socialization, women have different strengths and weaknesses than do men in communication and in negotiating their needs and concerns to partners about sex (Cline & McKenzie, 1994). In our society, women are seen as more expressive and communicative than men, and they may conceptualize intimacy in terms of being able and willing to communicate openly with a partner. Men, on the other hand, are taught to value action over expression, to be assertive, and to take risks. In sexual situations, these patterns may be quite detrimental for women seeking to exercise choice about sexual activity. Cline and McKenzie found that women are more likely to initiate discussions with partners about AIDS and condom use, and more likely to see themselves as vulnerable to disease, while men are more likely than women to take risks such as engaging in sexual activity with a greater number of partners.

Worth (1989) found that women's lack of power in their relationships with men, particularly regarding sexual practices and economic concerns, was among the reasons women gave for engaging in risky behaviors related to HIV. Women also reported they do not insist on using condoms because of the fear that their partners will think they are sexually promiscuous.

For some women, pressure from a partner to have unprotected sex sometimes escalates into violence. Biglan et al. (1995) examined whether coercion played a part in the high-risk sexual behavior of women. They defined behavior precipitated by coercion as any behavior "prompted by the aversive behavior of another" (p. 550), but found that the range of aversive behaviors experienced by women in such situations included everything from verbal intimidation to physical violence. Their study included five samples of women: Sample 1 was a group of 22 adolescents ranging in age from 15 to 19 who were sexually active; Samples 2 and 3 were two groups of 276 women from clinics where they were being treated for STDs; Sample 4 included 51 homeless women who were living on the street; and Sample 5 consisted of a group of 51 female college students.

When asked whether they had ever been forced to have sex, a proportion of women from each sample reported they had been forced, in the following percentages (Biglan et al., 1995): 41.7 percent of the adolescents in Sample 1; 46 percent of clinic patients in Sample 2; 39.1

percent of clinic patients in Sample 3; 68 percent of homeless women in Sample 4; and 22.4 percent of college women in Sample 5.

Although the college women (in Sample 5) appeared to be at the lowest risk, almost one-quarter of them had been forced to have sex as often as one to ten times (mean = 2.7 times). The majority of homeless women living on the street (Sample 4) had experienced forced sex (mean = 13.61 instances), some as many as 41 times during their lives (Biglan et al. 1995).

Besides being forced to have sex, women in this study reported having been coerced by men to have intercourse in other ways (Biglan et al., 1995). For example, 62.2 percent of one of the groups of women being seen at a clinic for treatment of STDs (Sample 2) said that they had intercourse with men when it was not their preference, because of frequent arguments related to having sex. Of the women from the clinic in Sample 2, 68.1 percent reported that some form of coercion by men was a factor that contributed to their involvement in high-risk sexual behavior. More than half of these women identified one or more situations involving coercion from a male partner that would have to be negotiated in order to adopt safer sex practices. One example of such a challenge included a "boyfriend getting frustrated and 'knocking me around'" (p. 563).

In addition to forced sexual encounters, Biglan et al. (1995) found a relationship between other forms of coercion and high-risk sexual behavior. They administered a measure of risky sexual behavior which included items such as number of partners, use of condoms, STD infection history, drug and alcohol use related to sexual activity, sex with partners who inject drugs, nonmonogomous sexual activity, and engaging in anal sex.

For subjects in all five samples, sexual coercion was highly correlated with risky sexual behavior and explained 21 percent of the variance in high-risk sexual behavior. Sexual coercion was significantly related to many of the individual items on the sexual risk-taking instrument: (1) the number of times respondents had sex over their life spans and also during the past year; (2) the total number of partners during the past year; and (3) the total number of nonmonogomous partners during the past year and during their lives. Coercion was also related to the use of alcohol and drugs when having sex, the number of partners who were not well known during the last year, anal sex, use of condoms and other types of birth control, and the number of STD infections over a lifetime.

SEXUAL ASSAULT

Sexual assault perpetrated by both strangers and acquaintances poses a significant threat to women's safety and health. Estimates of prevalence rates vary, but may be 20 percent or higher (Koss, 1993). The psychological aftermath of rape can last for years, sometimes for a lifetime, and is manifested as a variety of symptoms and disorders (Resick, 1993). Among the types of psychopathology found as consequences of rape are PTSD, depression, fear and anxiety, and impairments in self-esteem and sexual functioning.

Perhaps PTSD offers the best conceptualization of the effects of sexual assault. In one study (Rothbaum, Foa, Murdock, Riggs, and Walsh, 1992), 95 women who had been raped were examined over a period of three months. Ninety-four percent of victims met the diagnostic criteria for PTSD one week after being raped. Thirty-five days after the assault, 65 percent continued to meet the criteria. After 12 weeks, 47 percent of the subjects still qualified for the diagnosis. Other researchers (Kilpatrick et al., 1987) have found that PTSD is more common among rape victims than victims of other types of crime, with approximately 60 percent of those experiencing rape suffering from PTSD at some point during their lives.

Bownes, O'Gorman, and Sayers (1991) found that in a sample of 51 women who had been raped, 70 percent had PTSD. Women who were raped by strangers, physically injured during the rape, or whose attackers used physical force or weapons were more likely to develop PTSD. Furthermore, they found that other psychological problems, including depression, anxiety, and guilt, were more prevalent among those subjects with PTSD. In fact, depression often cooccurs with PTSD as a result of rape. In one study of rape victims (Cassiday, McNally, and Zeitlin, 1992), those with PTSD had the highest levels of depression.

Depression experienced as an outcome of rape seems to remain problematic over a period of years. Individuals with a history of having been raped (an average of 21.9 years earlier) were significantly more depressed than those who had not been raped (Kilpatrick et al., 1987). In a more recent study, Kilpatrick, Edmunds, and Seymour (1992) found that, of 507 rape victims, 21 percent were depressed at the time the survey was conducted and 30 percent had suffered an episode of major depression at some point during their lives. These figures are compared to a current rate of depression of 6 percent and a rate of 10 percent for depression over the course of their lives for women who had not been raped. In this study, 33 percent of the rape victims reported having considered suicide and 13 percent had attempted suicide, compared to subjects who had not experienced rape, who reported rates of 8 percent for considering suicide and 1 percent for attempting suicide.

Confounding these sexual assault outcomes is the finding from studies of sexual abuse which indicate that victims of childhood sexual abuse are more likely to be victims of sexual assault in adulthood (Kluft, 1990a). Dissociation appears to be a primary mediator between the childhood history of abuse and later victimization (Becker-Lausen et al., 1995; Kluft, 1990a). Thus, the symptomatology associated with rape may be confounded in some victims by psychopathology outcomes related to childhood histories of maltreatment.

Similarly, rape victims also have been found to experience subsequent difficulties with sexual functioning, which has also been identified as a major outcome related to childhood sexual abuse (Browne & Finkelhor, 1986). Another study (Becker, Skinner, Abel, & Chichon, 1986) found that 58.6 percent of female victims of sexual assault reported some type of sexual dysfunction, and 71 percent linked the dysfunction with the assault experience. The effects may be more damaging for women who are not regularly sexually active before the rape. Ellis, Calhoun, and Atkeson (1980) found that 43 percent of the women in their study who had been sexually active before being assaulted were avoiding sexual contact one month after the attack, but had resumed their previous levels of sexual activity within a year. Women who had been less sexually active before the assault were continuing to avoid sexual contact one year later.

Acquaintance or date rape appears to result in psychological disturbance as well. Shapiro and Schwarz (1997) found that college women who had been date-raped showed higher levels of indicators of trauma, including intrusive and dissociative symptoms, as well as sexual problems, when compared to college women who had not been raped. They also scored lower on a measure of sexual self-esteem. Other studies have indicated that victims of acquaintance rape are less likely to have reported the rape (Koss, Dinero, Seibel, & Cox, 1988), more likely than other rape victims to delay seeking treatment, and less likely to have defended themselves during the attack (Stewart et al., 1987).

HISTORY OF CHILD MALTREATMENT

As noted above, a childhood history of maltreatment, particularly sexual abuse, may confound some of the findings regarding outcomes of adult sexual assault. Van der Kolk (1996) suggests that victims of child abuse typically do not learn to regulate emotion and impulses as other children do. One of the consequences of this deficit is the lack of control of sexual impulses in adulthood. Briere (1992) describes this behavior as a "consciously or unconsciously chosen coping mechanism invoked to modulate painful internal experience" (pp. 67–68).

The relationship between child abuse and dissociation is well documented (Briere & Runtz, 1988; Nash, Hulsey, Sexton, Harralson, & Lambert, 1993). Dissociation (van der Kolk, 1996), which is common among abused children and adults with a history of child abuse, is the phenomenon of feeling detached from oneself and perceiving one's own experiences from a distant point of view. Gleeson (1996) also found a significant relationship between dissociation and a history of child maltreatment, and she further found that higher levels of dissociation were related to lower levels of knowledge about HIV and its transmission.

Children often use dissociation as a defense against the intense stress of child abuse (van der Kolk, 1996). While this mechanism helps to deal with the trauma of abuse while it is occurring, it is often generalized as a way of coping with stressful life situations. As a result, individuals who suffer trauma are often unable to discriminate real threat from harmless events. It is common for these individuals to miss the cues that might alert them to potentially dangerous situations. Because of the tendency to tune out the environment, they fail to notice events that others would interpret as signals of danger (Becker-Lausen et al., 1995; Kluft, 1990a):

> It was characteristic of these [dissociative] patients that they experienced extreme difficulty in perceiving and reacting to danger signals appropriately. It was heartbreaking to find that many of those who had been raped had in their minds useful but inaccessible data that would have allowed them to perceive the circumstances under which they had been raped as dangerous, and appropriate to avoid. However, these data were dissociated along with the recollection of the incidents in the course of which they had been learned. (Kluft, 1990a, p. 169)

Empirical studies have shown that sexual abuse victims are more likely than others to be raped later. Russell (1986) found that, of a sample of 930 women, at least 33 percent of those who had been sexually abused as children had later been raped, while, in a comparison group who had not been abused, just 17 percent had been raped. Miller et al. (1978) found that 18 percent of women who had been raped more that once were also victims of incest, compared to 4 percent of women who had been raped once.

Child sexual abuse is also believed to affect sexual activity in adulthood. Women who had been sexually abused often become sexually active at an earlier age (Briere, 1992; Wyatt, Newcomb, & Riederle, 1993). Studies have shown that women who were sexually abused as children tend to have their first sexual experiences earlier than women who did not experience child sexual abuse (Runtz & Briere, 1986).

Victims of sexual abuse are sometimes described as engaging in more high-risk sexual behavior as adults and adolescents. For example, women who were sexually abused in childhood reported a greater number of sexual partners and sexual relationships of shorter duration in adolescence (Wyatt, 1988). According to Erickson and Rapkin (1991), adolescents with histories of child sexual abuse and other unwanted sexual experiences were more likely to report being sexually active and to have had an STD. They were also less likely to report using contraceptives. Van der Kolk (1989) suggests such behaviors may result from what Freud (1920/1964) called the "compulsion to repeat" the trauma, a phenomenon whereby the victim must act out events of the past repeatedly in an attempt to reduce the anxiety associated with an initial, similar event.

However, Browne and Finkelhor (1986) caution that self-reported findings related to sexual activity might be confounded due to abuse victims' negative self-attributions, citing a study by Fromuth (1983), in which victims of sexual abuse did not differ from controls in the number of sexual partners they had, only in their tendencies to define their own behavior as "promiscuous." Likewise, in Gleeson's (1996) study, no relationship was found between subjects' reported number of sexual partners and their history of child abuse.

However, the research suggests that there may be a link between child sexual abuse and later prostitution. Among a sample of 136 prostitutes, 55 percent reported childhood sexual abuse by someone at least 10 years older than themselves (James & Meyerding, 1977). Sixty-five percent of the adolescents in this sample reported having been forced to have sex before age 16. In a study by Bagley and Young (1987), 73 percent of a group of former prostitutes reported being sexually abused as children.

DRUG USE AND RISKY SEXUAL BEHAVIOR

Injection drug use has been a major cause of HIV infection of women throughout the AIDS epidemic (Kalichman, 1995). Until 1992, injection drug use was the leading cause of women becoming infected with HIV. An estimated 40 percent of injection drug users share needles in a variety of contexts. Needles may be shared with new users who are being taught how to inject drugs. Users also rent needles to others in exchange for money used to purchase drugs. Drug users may not take needles with them when they leave home for fear of being arrested, and may instead use needles that belong to others to inject drugs when they are away from home.

Women are placed at risk not only by their own drug use, but also through sex with partners who are injection drug users. Recently, crack use has also been identified as a kind of drug use that increases risky sexual behavior, particularly among women. Inciardi (1995) examined the relationship between crack use and HIV risk, noting that in the late 1980s, it was believed that smoking crack was a safer alternative (i.e., related to HIV risk) to the use of cocaine by injection. However, because crack users often exchange sex for the drug, they are likely to have unprotected sex with a large number of partners (Inciardi, 1995). Later research has indicated that HIV infection risk is at least as high among crack users as among injection drug users and that HIV is more likely to be spread by women who trade sex for crack than by women who used cocaine or heroin.

Inciardi's (1995) study consisted of interviews with 17 men and 35 women who had used crack at least three days per week for the 30-day period prior to the study, and who had exchanged sex for crack or for money to purchase crack. The interview examined drug use, sexual practices, and knowledge about HIV. The study revealed that while both men and women engaged in frequent and varied sexual activities, women engaged in sex more often than men. Thirty-one of the 35 female subjects reported having had 100 or more male partners during the last 30 days. Thirty-nine percent reportedly had had vaginal intercourse more than 50 times, 57 percent reported having oral sex more than 50 times, and 20 percent indicated that they had engaged in anal sex during the 30 days prior to the study.

Condom use was also low among these women (Inciardi, 1995). Twenty-three percent indicated they had always used condoms during vaginal intercourse, while only 14 percent consistently used condoms during oral sex. Out of the seven women who had had anal sex, only two had used condoms.

These women had misconceptions about HIV and its transmission (Inciardi, 1995). Forty-three percent believed that 90 percent of people in the United States who have AIDS are gay. Eighty-six percent believed that one can become infected with HIV by kissing, sneezing, or sharing food. Eighty-six percent believed that a person who becomes infected with HIV feels ill immediately. However, 92 percent reported at least a fairly high degree of concern about AIDS and 91 percent knew that using condoms could prevent HIV infection.

This study also revealed that women who exchange sex for crack are probably at higher risk for HIV infection than are prostitutes (Inciardi, 1995). Prostitutes are believed to have fewer sex partners overall. In this study, prostitutes reported having three to six sexual contacts per day on 15 to 30 days out of the month. Prostitutes are more likely to guard against STDs and other dangers due to information gained from more experienced prostitutes or from their pimps. The atmosphere in crack houses perhaps also accounts for the difference in risk. Women who engage in sex for drugs often have sex in crack houses. They may binge on crack for several days at a time, getting high many times per day. Obtaining crack is a primary motivator for these women and often they are powerless over the demands of others.

MOTHERS OF INFANTS BORN WITH HIV

HIV can be transmitted from mother to child in several ways (Kalichman, 1995). Most frequently, HIV antibodies are passed from the mother to the fetus in utero through the placenta. Typically, this occurs during the second or third trimester of pregnancy. Another method of transmission is through the infant's contact at birth with the mother's infected blood or vaginal fluid. Because the virus is present in the breast milk of an infected mother, HIV may be passed from mother to infant through breast-feeding.

Each year in the United States, approximately 6000 HIV-infected women give birth (Kalichman, 1995). Between 20 percent and 40 percent of those infants are born with HIV. Women who have recently been infected and those who are in a more advanced stage of HIV infection are most likely to transmit the virus to their children. The risk for transmission may be reduced if the mother is treated with an antiretroviral medication such as zidovudine, commonly known as AZT.

Children born with HIV do not survive as long as HIV-infected adults do (Kalichman, 1995). They begin to show symptoms of HIV between 8 and 10 months of age. In addition, they are more susceptible to disease in general than other children because of their reduced immune function. These children are likely to show failure to thrive and may show delays in reaching developmental milestones, as well as difficulty in maintaining such milestones. Children with HIV are more likely than adults to develop AIDS dementia complex, a disease that has devastating effects on cognitive and motor abilities. In its most advanced stage, AIDS dementia complex induces a vegetative state, paraplegia, and mutism.

Children of HIV mothers also run the risk of being orphaned due to AIDS; often these children are born to parents who are both HIV positive. Mothers face not only the difficulty of dealing with their illness, but must also cope with fears about their children's future. These women are likely to be poor and to have limited access to health care and other resources that are particularly vital to their survival and well-being.

Mothers who give birth to HIV-infected children are most likely to have contracted the virus through injection drug use or through heterosexual contact (Rogers & Kilbourne, 1992). Babies whose mothers are drug users face not only the problems associated with HIV infection, but problems related to drug addiction as well. Newborns infected with HIV are most likely to have been born to poor, ethnic minority women who live in the inner city.

FETAL EFFECTS OF ALCOHOL USE

Maternal alcohol consumption during pregnancy is related to a pattern of birth defects called fetal alcohol syndrome (FAS). FAS causes a variety of abnormalities in infants (Manteuffel, 1996), including brain abnormalities and mental retardation. Children with FAS may suffer from hyperactivity, slowed reaction times, and attention, behavior, and perceptual problems.

FAS seems to be related to patterns of heavy drinking, involving blood alcohol levels above 0.1 percent, rather than to more moderate consumption of alcohol during pregnancy (Abel, 1996). However, because research on this problem leaves many questions unanswered, many experts advise pregnant women to avoid all alcohol.

Research is underway to determine how alcohol consumption at different stages of pregnancy are related to specific kinds of defects (Maier, Chen, & West, 1996). Currently, it is believed that the facial defects associated with FAS are caused by alcohol consumption around the time of conception and in the first trimester of pregnancy. Women who drink heavily and are considering pregnancy are advised to adjust their alcohol consumption to minimize this risk. Hankin (1996) advises targeting women over 30 who drink and become pregnant for FAS awareness, because this population has been found to be less influenced than younger women by warning labels about birth defects on alcoholic beverages.

PSYCHOLOGICAL CONSEQUENCES
OF ABORTION

Mental health experts differ widely in their opinions about the severity of the psychological sequelae of abortion. The quality of existing research in this area is also in question. Wilmoth et al. (1992) raise objections regarding the quality of instruments used, the selection of subjects, attrition of subjects from samples, the imprecise definition of constructs being studied, and the lack of comparison groups. These authors emphasize the political nature of this area of study as well.

Wilmoth et al. (1992) describe the range of opinions on the psychological effects of abortion as a "continuum" (p. 39). At one end, they place the work of Adler (1992; also see Adler et al., 1990), who maintains that severe psychological problems resulting from abortion are uncommon. Adler suggests that the circumstances surrounding a pregnancy and its termination are important factors which should be examined in connection with potential psychological effects. At the other end of the continuum are Speckhard and Rue (1992), authors who propose that many women experience considerable negative psychological aftereffects of abortion.

Speckhard and Rue (1992) describe these symptoms as a syndrome that resembles PTSD, which they refer to as Postabortion Syndrome or PAS. PAS is defined by the following criteria: (1) having experienced an abortion and interpreted this experience as traumatic; (2) reexperiencing the abortion involuntarily, such as through flashbacks or nightmares; (3) a diminished ability to relate to others and the environment due to attempts to avoid painful memories and negative affect related to the abortion; (4) other related psychological symptoms not experienced before the abortion.

Two variations on the psychological consequences of abortion, Postabortion Distress (PAD) and Postabortion Psychosis (PAP), are proposed by Speckhard and Rue (1992). Like PAS, neither of these syndromes is accepted by the American Psychiatric Association as a psychological disorder, but each may be useful for understanding the possible range of psychological problems that may result from abortion. PAD involves some difficulty with the aftermath of abortion, but is less severe than the trauma that occurs with PAS. The authors liken

PAD to a type of adjustment disorder that is characterized by physical and emotional distress related to the pregnancy or abortion, a sense of loss following the abortion, and psychological conflict as a result of having had the abortion.

PAP is a more severe and less common outcome than PAS and involves thought disorder or a serious emotional disturbance caused by the abortion (Speckhard & Rue, 1992). Symptoms of PAP include significant levels of depression, guilt, and hallucinations, as well as fear related to having others know about the abortion.

INTERVENTIONS

Many of the problems discussed in this chapter can be grouped in terms of their psychological components and the type of intervention that would be most useful in addressing them. Below are some of these intervention approaches. Problems resulting from lack of awareness of risk involving unsafe sex practices can be treated with psychoeducational programs that include assertiveness skills and hands-on practice in dealing with awkward situations. Interventions based on Fisher and Fisher's (1992) IMB model are likely to be successful. A treatment for PTSD is described as a strategy for problems resulting in trauma, such as sexual assault.

Interventions for Safer Sex

While adequate knowledge about these issues is essential, women also need behavioral skills that will allow them to act in accord with the knowledge they possess. In addition, societal attitudes related to power issues between men and women must change in order for women to be effective in controlling sexual situations. Cline and McKenzie (1994) suggest that, while most existing HIV prevention programs stress the idea that it is important for partners to talk to one another about their past sexual partners and the use of condoms (Cline, 1991), merely talking about these issues is insufficient to prevent the spread of HIV. They stress that condom use should be the outcome of such discussions, and women should anticipate resistance from men related to discussing AIDS.

These authors (Cline & McKenzie, 1994) suggest a strategy for changing women's attitudes about condom use which includes framing a male partner's willingness to use condoms as a "caring" behavior (p. 334). Men also should be given the message that women will perceive a man's willingness to use a condom as a positive behavior and, therefore, will not be offended by a man's wish to use a condom. Stressing that safe sex is more pleasurable because of the sense of being protected from negative outcomes is another useful strategy.

Because women report embarrassment about buying condoms, Cline and McKenzie (1994) suggest making condoms easier for women to buy anonymously. Women should also be given the message that buying condoms is a positive action. Role-play exercises can be used to help women practice buying condoms.

The effectiveness of a one-session informational intervention was compared to a multiple-session, skills-training intervention designed to promote safe sex practices among a group of 91 women in methadone treatment (el Bassel & Schilling, 1992). Immediately following the intervention, women in the skills-training condition who reported being sexually active were found to be more likely to discuss safe sex practices and to carry and use condoms than were sexually active members of the information-only intervention. In addition, members of the skills-training group were more likely to believe that AIDS is preventable and to be interested in obtaining information about AIDS, and less likely to consider HIV infection to be a matter of luck. After 15 months, the skills-training group continued to feel more at ease in discussing safe sex practices and still believed that AIDS is preventable. However, they were more likely than controls to consider HIV infection a matter of luck and were no more likely than controls to carry condoms.

Sikkema, Winett, and Lombard (1995) used a behavioral intervention which taught participants "sexual assertiveness." Female college students developed assertiveness skills in a group setting led by a female graduate student. The group was presented with a scenario which might result in a high-risk sexual behavior. Adaptive responses were modeled for the group. Such responses consisted of declining to participate in the risky sexual behavior suggested by the partner, as well as explaining why the request was unacceptable and the offering of a safer activity. Participants had the opportunity to practice responding in such situations, and group discussion addressed the efficacy of such responses. Each participant received 40 condoms, distributed to each group member during the last two sessions.

Based on these studies, an effective group intervention for women should consist of the following components:

1. Women should receive factual information about AIDS and other STDs, including how the HIV virus is transmitted and the specific danger to women (which is often understated).

2. Women should be presented with convincing arguments for using condoms and encouraged to discuss their reservations regarding the implications of condom use, including their own values and expected responses of partners.

3. Objections to condom use should be challenged. Condom use should be presented as an act of consideration for one's partner as well as a safeguard of one's own life and health.

4. Group members should be taught assertive communication skills tailored to use in situations involving negotiations about sex.

5. Group members should role-play negotiating safe sex practices with partners. Role-play is an especially important activity since many women may not be skilled in being assertive with men in sexual situations.

Interventions should also address differences in ethnicity. Wyatt and Riederle (1994) suggest that, in traditional cultures, a woman may draw most of her sense of self-worth from her role as a mother. The authors recommend targeting these women with the message that practicing safe sex is a way to care for their families. For women who have been socialized to see themselves and their own lives as inconsequential, the importance of protecting their children could be a more powerful motivator.

Overall, safe sex interventions for women should stress the fact that using condoms and refusing high-risk behaviors are essentially no less than matters of life and death in today's society. Women must understand that they are powerful agents and that they are ultimately responsible for their health and for protecting their unborn children from STDs.

Intervention for Trauma

Calhoun and Resick (1993) outline a technique called cognitive processing therapy, which was designed for the treatment of PTSD resulting from rape (Resick & Schnicke, 1992). Cognitive processing therapy consists of two main components. One aspect involves desensitization related to the traumatic event. This is accomplished by having the client write about the event while remembering and including the affect associated with the event at the time that it occurred. These written accounts are then read aloud by the client during sessions. The other component of this treatment involves cognitive restructuring and consists of helping the client distinguish how the event has affected her beliefs about herself, other people, and the world, and how these changed beliefs conflict with preexisting schemas regarding issues such as personal safety, trust of others, and personal relationships. Therapy focuses on challenging these new, maladaptive beliefs, resolving the trauma experience, and reestablishing a more positive view of oneself and the world. Cognitive processing therapy may be conducted individually or in a group setting. Calhoun and Resick (1993) suggest that, for the treatment of rape victims, the social support provided in a group setting often serves to reduce self-blame and to bolster the self-esteem of victims. A typical structure for the use of cognitive processing therapy is presented below (Calhoun & Resick, 1993).

In the first few sessions, clients are informed of the treatment rationale. For example, explanations of how the traumatic event might have upset the client's belief system are proposed. Clients are informed that major goals of treatment are (1) to work through the emotion associated with the rape; and (2) to restore a healthy perspective about the self and others. Clients are given a homework assignment to write about the traumatic event and its meaning for them. (For example, Calhoun and Resick give an example of a client who blames herself for being raped. She is asked to write about the experience, including details of how it affects her beliefs about herself and other people, particularly in terms of safety, power, and intimacy.)

The client is asked to read her homework during a session, so that the therapist can help her identify what Calhoun and Resick (1993) call "stuck points," i.e., points of conflict between maladaptive beliefs resulting from the trauma and previously held beliefs. Homework consists of identifying events that occurred, determining the client's beliefs about the events, and labeling the emotions resulting from the beliefs.

Maladaptive beliefs about the events are confronted and challenged during sessions. The client is encouraged to explore alternative meanings for the events that have been identified, with a goal of the alternative meanings leading to more adaptive emotional responses. For example, a woman who identifies an event by the fact that she was raped by an armed man and that she did not struggle may have a corresponding belief that the rape was her fault. The related emotional response may be guilt. However, an alternative belief about this event would be that to avoid struggling with an armed attacker was the safest course of action, and that she may have protected her life by not resisting. The emotional response could then be a more positive one, e.g., feeling she was smart or courageous. The client is given five modules written by Resick and Schnicke (1993) focusing on the topics of safety, trust, power, esteem, and intimacy. The modules examine the effects of maladaptive beliefs in these areas and include recommended alternatives.

Near the end of treatment, the client is asked to rewrite her account of the rape and read it aloud during a session. The client and therapist review the progress since the first writing exercise. Calhoun and Resick (1993) suggest 12 sessions for this treatment.

SUMMARY AND CONCLUSIONS

In this chapter we have reviewed research which highlights the unique problems of women with regard to their involvement in high-risk sexual behavior and its outcomes. Intimidation, coercion, and violence by partners often make it problematic for women to engage in protective behaviors around sexual activity. Traumatic experiences resulting from sexual assault, sometimes compounded by childhood experiences of abuse, may lead to sequelae which make it difficult for a woman to respond effectively in risky situations. Dissociation, particularly, has been shown to contribute to this increased vulnerability to revictimization.

As we have discussed in this chapter, use of alcohol and other drugs greatly increases high-risk sexual behavior. Crack house sex in exchange for drugs, for example, has been found to be more hazardous for women, with regard to HIV infection, than injection drug use. Women's behavior also poses special risks to their children. For example, HIV-positive mothers may pass the virus on to their offspring, and they also may leave their children orphaned. Use of alcohol and other drugs may leave their children seriously compromised at birth. Alcohol has been associated with the worst outcomes in this regard.

Abortion, which eliminates the potential for these negative birth outcomes, may be psychologically difficult for some women, especially those who are vulnerable to depression and other posttraumatic stress symptoms. However, for many women abortion does not appear to create any psychological symptomatology. Unfortunately, what we know about the vulnerabilities associated with a history of childhood maltreatment and subsequent negative life outcomes, including substance abuse, psychopathology, prostitution, and revictimization, would indicate that those women most likely to engage in some of these hazardous behaviors are also the women most likely to find abortion upsetting and stressful. Treatment of traumatic symptoms that empowers women to take greater control of their lives may ultimately reduce some of these risk factors.

SUGGESTIONS FOR INTERVENTIONS

Basics of intervention approaches were presented in this chapter. These strategies must be incorporated into a wide range of intervention programs, including those for substance abuse, for problematic parenting, and for battered women. Below we discuss which types of strategies are likely to be effective.

Successful Strategies

The most successful strategies are likely to incorporate the elements of Fisher and Fisher's (1992) IMB model. This model suggests a combination of education presented in such a way that individuals understand the risks they face and are convinced to take appropriate action as well as skills training that teaches effective responses one might use in risky situations. See Chapter 3 for more information on this model.

Skills training is a particularly important component of interventions for women. Role-playing in group settings has been particularly effective in developing competence and, consequently, changing behavior.

Strategies that May Succeed

Changing perceptions about condom use among women could result in positive behavior change. Interventions that associate condom use with responsibility and consideration for one's partner rather than with promiscuity or lack of trust may be beneficial. Making condoms easier to purchase anonymously could increase women's willingness to buy and use them.

Programs that teach women to be assertive in their relationships with men may be successful. However, it is unreasonable to expect that women who find themselves in coercive, manipulative, or violent relationships will be able to use such training to great advantage.

Unsuccessful Strategies

Interventions that only impart information about the risks of unsafe sex probably do not result in substantial behavior change. Women need to understand their level of risk and acquire skills to address these risks. Interventions that stress communication between partners are also likely to fail. Communication about risk is insufficient to ensure behavior change, particularly in relationships where women may be less powerful than their male partners.

6

Guidelines for Intervention, III
Gay Men and Bisexuals

INTERVENTION EFFORTS IN THE GAY COMMUNITY

In this chapter, factors affecting the gay community are addressed. Prevention and intervention outcomes are presented first, followed by some of the key issues that affect sexual risk-taking, such as the use of alcohol and other drugs, trauma history, partner coercion, grief, and loss. Issues that arise in treatment with clients who are living with AIDS or who are partners of HIV-infected individuals are presented. Death, dying, and grief in the gay community are also discussed.

INTRODUCTION

Because AIDS was first identified in gay men, much of the research and prevention work has been carried out with this population. Behavioral research initially targeted the identification of high-risk sexual practices in the gay community, resulting in the finding that gay men engaged in a range of sexual activities with a diversity of sexual partners (Cochran, de Leeuw, & Mays, 1995). Out of these early studies, guidelines for the adoption of safer sexual practices were developed. For gay men, these practices include using condoms for anal intercourse as well as reducing the frequency of engaging in anal intercourse.

Despite widespread acceptance of these behavioral adaptations, gay and bisexual men still comprise a large proportion of AIDS cases in the United States. In June 1994, gay and bisexual men represented 59 percent of all adolescent and adult AIDS cases in the United States, and they constituted half of all new cases of AIDS and 75 percent of new male cases of AIDS reported between July 1993 to June 1994 (Meyer & Dean, 1995).

Most of the research with gay and bisexual men has been conducted in major urban centers, such as San Francisco and New York, with relatively few studies investigating patterns of sexual risk-taking among gay men in less populated areas (Kelly et al., 1995).

In the 1990s, studies of these urban populations have shown the alarming reemergence of a trend toward increasing rates of high-risk sexual behavior, particularly among younger gay and bisexual men (Meyer & Dean, 1995). Furthermore, when research has been undertaken with gay men in smaller communities, the findings indicate these men also may be at great risk, particularly those who are younger or less educated (Kelly et al., 1995).

PREVENTION AND INTERVENTION

Behavioral Changes over Time

Substantial reductions in risky sexual behavior within the gay community have been identified in numerous studies, yet by the mid-1990s, concern was growing that these changes were not being sustained (Dawson et al., 1994). As this concern has come to light, researchers have increasingly studied factors associated with maintaining changes over time.

By 1991, researchers were reporting that gay men had significantly reduced their high-risk sexual behavior (Kelly & Murphy, 1991). Two longitudinal surveys of more than 1000 gay men in San Francisco showed substantial increases in condom use over time, which appeared to be unaffected by biases related to subjects who dropped out of the study or other selection factors (Catania et al., 1991). In a study of bar patrons in San Francisco, 593 gay men were compared to 314 heterosexual men and 437 heterosexual women (McKusick,

Hoff, Stall, & Coates, 1991). Results indicated gay men were more likely than heterosexual subjects to use condoms and to obtain an HIV antibody test; however, heterosexuals were more likely to report fewer sexual partners and to have attempted to determine characteristics of potential partners by using interview strategies.

Despite these encouraging changes in behavior, researchers were well aware that individuals within these populations varied considerably in their acceptance of safer sex practices, their ability to implement them, and their maintenance of these changes over time. In the longitudinal study conducted in San Francisco by Catania and colleagues (1991), gay men who reported always using condoms had higher levels of informal social support and more positive expectations about personal and interpersonal effects of condom use. They were also more likely to be HIV *positive* than men who reported intermittent or no condom use, indicating prosocial reasons may play an important role in these decisions.

Risk Factors

In order to study specific factors associated with the inability to sustain sexual behavior changes, Kelly, St. Lawrence, and Brasfield (1991) followed 68 gay men for 16 months after they attended AIDS prevention sessions. Relapse of high-risk sexual behavior was associated with the following characteristics: younger age; beginning at an earlier age to engage in unprotected, receptive, anal intercourse often and with many partners; having had more sexual partners; reinforcement values related to high-risk sexual practices and use of condoms; being intoxicated prior to sex; lower levels of reported depression; beliefs related to HIV infection which reflect an external locus of control (i.e., becoming infected is a matter of luck or chance); and disclosure of sexual orientation (i.e., "coming out" as a gay man). Based on these characteristics, Kelly and colleagues were able to correctly classify 86 percent of the sample as either in maintenance or in relapse with regard to their safer sex practices, using a discriminant function analysis statistical technique.

Inconsistent AIDS prevention behaviors among gay men have also been linked to a number of cognitive distortions, including faulty beliefs that one is at low risk of HIV infection and a tendency to explain risky sexual behavior as atypical and situational, thereby diminishing the degree to which the individual views his own behavior as putting him at risk (Offir, Fisher, Williams, & Fisher, 1993). In addition, Martin (1993) found high-risk behavior was associated with passive coping styles in a sample of 324 gay men. Subjects were more likely to reduce risky behaviors when they believed they could change or could prevent AIDS, and when they used active coping styles such as seeking social support.

As the 1990s unfolded, concern began to grow for the gay community, as studies revealed that some younger gay men were not reporting the same level of safer sexual practices as their older counterparts. For example, among 61 gay male college students under age 25, few had made major changes in their sexual behavior to prevent the risk of HIV infection, although only 8 percent said they were not worried about the risk (D'Augelli, 1992b). Most of these subjects had not instituted the effective practices reported by older generations of gay men (such as condom use), and they reported relying primarily on reduced numbers of partners and being selective in their choice of partners as a means of preventing HIV infection.

Cultural Factors of Risk

Also in the 1990s, the need to focus attention on cultural factors of risk began to be recognized. For example, black gay men were perceived to be at a particular disadvantage, because of the combination of racist and homophobic attitudes in the community at large (Icard, Schilling, el Bassel, & Young, 1992). The emphasis on AIDS in the gay community, which is predominantly white, may have created a misperception that HIV is a problem for the white community only. For gay and bisexual men, African Americans, Latinos, and women, some researchers have suggested that being a member of more than one of these groups (e.g., minority women, gay minority men) adds to the difficulties of implementing prevention strategies, because of the cumulative effects of stigma and discrimination for these groups (Croteau, Nero, & Prosser, 1993). Specific cultural issues are discussed in greater detail in Chapter 4.

High-risk sexual behavior has been found to be considerably more prevalent among African-American gay and bisexual men compared to their white counterparts. In one of the first studies of nonwhite homosexual men, Peterson and colleagues (1992) found that 52 percent of the 250 gay and bisexual African-American subjects interviewed in the San Francisco Bay Area in 1990 reported having unprotected anal intercourse in the prior six months, compared to 15 to 20 percent of their white counterparts in San Francisco in 1988 who admitted to engaging in this behavior. African-American gay and bisexual men were more likely to have engaged in this high-risk practice if they were low income, if they had used injection drugs, and/or if they had been paid for the sexual activity.

These outcomes occurred despite the fact that these men did perceive themselves to be at risk for HIV infection, indicating that educational campaigns to increase perceptions of risk were not sufficient to change high-risk behavior in this population. Peterson and colleagues (1992) suggest instead that building skills, shifting norms, and increasing awareness of condoms' ability to prevent disease all are strategies to be used with this population. In addition, outreach to impact the most vulnerable segments of the population will be necessary to change high-risk behaviors.

A more recent study employed statistical techniques (i.e., latent structural models) that allow for an examination of common underlying patterns with samples representing diverse populations, in order to improve prediction of behavior (Cochran et al., 1995). This study suggests there may be a commonality of risk factors across cultural groups. With a sample of 343 predominantly white gay men who attended a workshop and a nationally recruited sample of 837 African-American gay men, researchers again found significantly higher rates of risky sexual behavior among the African-American men. However, as predicted, they also found a single, unifying pattern of behaviors related to sexual risk-taking in both samples, with differences primarily occurring in the rates at which these behaviors are carried out within each population. Although these findings do not necessarily indicate that motivational, decision-making, or social influence factors are similar for different ethnic groups, they do suggest that there may be striking commonalities across cultures which are relevant for targeted prevention programs.

Within cultural groups, individual differences also exist. In a study of 200 gay, bisexual, and transvestite men in Juarez, Mexico,

Ramirez and colleagues (Ramirez, Suarez, de la Rosa, Castro, & Zimmerman, 1994) again found levels of AIDS knowledge were high, but behaviors did not necessarily reflect information levels. Receptive anal and oral sexual activity was more common among gay men than among bisexual men; however, bisexual men were more likely than gay men to practice insertive anal intercourse. Higher risk was associated with lower occupational levels, as well as with sexual partners met on the street, compared to those met in bars or discos. Contrary to findings in predominantly white U.S. samples (e.g., D'Augelli, 1992b), older subjects in this Mexican sample were *less* likely to use condoms than younger subjects. Subjects with *more* sexual partners used condoms *less* often than those with fewer partners.

Nonurban Populations

In their study of nearly 6000 men in gay bars in 16 smaller U.S. cities, Kelly and colleagues (1995) found that 27 percent of these men admitted anonymously that they had engaged in unprotected anal intercourse during the prior two months. Those who engaged in this behavior were more likely to report greater numbers of partners, lower levels of intention to use condoms, beliefs that they were personally at greater risk, and beliefs that one's peers did not hold safer sex as a normative behavior. Subjects reporting high-risk behavior were also younger and less educated, leading the researchers to suggest that it may be beneficial to design interventions targeting younger and less educated gay men, particularly in smaller communities.

Bisexuals

Bisexual men may also need interventions specifically designed for them. In a study of 1180 gay men and 136 bisexual men (Heckman et al., 1995), the bisexual subjects anonymously reported less intention to use condoms, higher rates of oral sex with males, greater numbers of oral sex partners, and greater perceptions that safer sex and avoidance of risky behaviors were not normative to their peer group, compared to gay men. Bisexual men also knew fewer individuals who were HIV positive. Among the bisexual men, 33 percent had, in the prior two months, engaged in unprotected anal intercourse, 17 percent with multiple partners. The authors recommend that interventions for bisexual men focus on changing normative expectations, increasing intentionality related to condom use, and on psychoeducation regarding HIV transmission and risky sexual behavior.

Studies with European Populations

Studies of risk factors among gay and bisexual men in Europe have revealed similar findings to U.S. studies; for example, increasingly high rates of infection outside urban centers (Hart et al., 1993). In a survey of more than 12,000 gay and bisexual men in eight European countries (Austria, Denmark, France, Germany, Great Britain, Italy, the Netherlands, and Switzerland), sexual behavior reported across these cultures was notably similar; however, risk management strategies varied considerably (Bochow et al., 1994). In countries where prevention campaigns targeting the gay community had been instituted early, risk-reduction strategies were the most prevalent. Reported rates of HIV-positive antibody tests ranged from fewer than 7 percent in East Germany, Great Britain, and Italy to 15 percent for Denmark and 17 percent for France. The majority of gay men in the survey reported multiple partners, but anal intercourse was more likely to occur in more stable relationships than between casual partners.

In a study of more than 1000 gay-identified, predominantly white men attending Gay Pride festivals between 1993 and 1995 in Great Britain, Hickson and colleagues (1996) found that, despite HIV prevention programs, levels of unprotected anal intercourse remained relatively unchanged. The authors concluded that high-risk sexual behavior may show considerable stability and resistance to change.

Other studies conducted with gay and/or bisexual men in Great Britain have found safer sexual behavior to be associated with acculturation to (i.e., identification with) the gay community (Seibt et al., 1995); a relationship between lifetime incidence of STDs and HIV positive status (Williams et al., 1996); and, contrary to some U.S. studies (e.g., Kelly et al., 1991), British researchers found *no* relationship between alcohol consumption and engaging in risky sexual behavior (Weatherburn et al., 1993).

Other Risk Factors

Studies in the 1990s have continued to explore factors associated with high-risk sexual behavior in gay men. In a study of 53 HIV-negative gay men in North Carolina, outside the urban centers of the AIDS epidemic, high-risk sexual behavior was found to be associated with a number of psychological factors (Perkins, Leserman, Murphy, & Evans, 1993). In this sample, 23.1 percent of the subjects were classified as engaging in high-risk sexual behavior, with 60 percent reporting low-risk behaviors and 17.3 percent categorized as moderately at risk by their behaviors. Higher risk behaviors were associated with higher rates of reported optimism and anger, with lower levels of emotional control, and with less acceptance as a gay man.

Perceptions of sexual control have also been identified as a factor in high-risk sexual practices among 108 HIV-positive and 48 HIV-negative gay men in New York City (Exner, Meyer-Bahlburg, & Ehrhardt, 1992). Reported difficulty controlling sexual behavior was associated with more sex partners, more lifetime and recent rates (i.e., past six months) of sexual encounters, more one-time and outside-the-home sexual partners, less monogamy, and with abstinance from sexual behavior in the past six months. Perceived difficulties with control were also related to greater drug use, to the use of cocaine or amyl nitrate during sexual activity, and to the tendency to engage in higher risk sexual behaviors. Those reporting lower perceived control were more likely to have engaged in receptive, ejaculatory anal intercourse than those who perceived themselves as having greater sexual control.

Finally, in Meyer and Dean's (1995) investigation of 174 young (age 18 to 24), gay men in New York City, about two-thirds of the sample engaged in receptive anal intercourse in each year of the two-year period of the study. One-third of the total sample had anal intercourse that was unprotected. However, the men who engaged in these behaviors were more likely to be in a relationship with their partner, and more likely to know this partner's HIV status. Similar to other studies, Meyer and Dean found that receptive anal intercourse was associated with use of alcohol and other drugs during sexual activity, earlier age of initial sexual experiences, and greater acculturation to the gay community.

About six percent of the sample were found to engage in extremely high-risk sex, i.e., unprotected, receptive anal intercourse with multiple sex partners. Meyer and Dean (1995) found qualitative differences between this small subset of the sample and the other subjects who sometimes engaged in high-risk sexual practices. Whereas mental health problems were not identifiably related to risky sexual behavior in the broader sample, the extremely high-risk subset had significantly greater drug use, higher rates of internalized homophobia, and more AIDS-related traumatic stress.

FACTORS AFFECTING INTERVENTION

Risk factors such as those described above often interfere with the effectiveness of intervention with the highest risk subgroups within the gay community (e.g., injection drug users). Significant risk factors include a history of maltreatment in childhood; abuse of alcohol and other drugs; personality issues; and partner coercion, intimidation, or violence.

Child Maltreatment History

Despite the explosion of research on child maltreatment, few studies have examined the implications of a child abuse history for gay men, particularly with regard to high-risk sexual practices. What literature exists in this area primarily presents either single-case, clinical examples (e.g., Millan & Caban, 1996) or theoretical perspectives, often with a treatment focus (e.g., Hoisen, 1993; Shernoff & Finnegan, 1991). The latter writings appear mostly in the chemical dependency literature.

As some authors have suggested, however, the issue of maltreatment is a complex one for the gay community, because it is confounded by the potential for verbal and physical abuse resulting from homophobia. For example, Savin-Williams (1994) notes that, among gay and bisexual youth, chronic stress results from the verbal and physical abuse they endure from both adults and peers. Thus, among gay youth, problems relevant to high-risk sexual behavior, such as substance abuse, running away, and prostitution may result, in part, from multiple forms of societal and institutionalized maltreatment.

These factors may increase the risk for gay youth of the relevant
negative outcomes which have been associated with maltreatment
within the family, including substance abuse, homelessness, prostitution, and the tendency to engage in frequent sexual activity with
multiple partners as a means of relieving abuse-related dysphoria
(Becker-Lausen & Gleeson, 1996; Briere, 1992; Rickel & Becker,
1997). However, the links between homophobia-related maltreatment
and these negative outcomes have yet to be empirically established
(Savin-Williams, 1994). Determining the effects of child abuse and
neglect as distinct from outcomes resulting from societal and institu-
tional abuse related to homophobia constitutes a challenging task for
future researchers. Clearly, both forms of maltreatment constitute
potentially traumatic experiences of childhood and adolescence.

Among the few studies examining child maltreatment history with
a gay population, Bartholow and colleagues' (1994) research involved
interviews with 1001 adult gay and bisexual men attending urban clinics
for STDs. Subjects (who were 73 percent white, 12 percent black, 12
percent Hispanic, and 4 percent Asian) were asked about childhood
sexual abuse experiences. About one-third of this sample (34 percent)
met the criteria for child sexual abuse, which included factors such as
age difference between sexual partners, anal penetration, and the use of
force. Outcomes were similar to studies of sexual abuse in other groups,
with a few findings that were specific to this population.

Similar to outcomes with other populations (Briere, 1992), a
reported history of sexual abuse was associated with higher rates of
substance use, depression, suicidal ideation or attempts, psychotherapy
treatment, psychiatric and substance use hospitalization, and a lack of
social support, compared to subjects who did not report a sexual abuse
history (Bartholow et al., 1994).

Furthermore, childhood sexual abuse reports were associated
with high-risk sexual behavior in these gay men. Men who reported
abuse histories were more likely to have engaged in unprotected anal
intercourse, receptive anal intercourse (with stable partners), and injection drug use (Bartholow et al., 1994). They were also twice as likely
to have been paid for sex. Abused Hispanic men were twice as likely
as black or white men to engage in receptive anal intercourse with their
steady partners. Given these high-risk behaviors, it is not surprising
that sexual abuse victims were significantly more likely to test positive

both for syphilis and for HIV infection (although this finding did not hold for other STDs, such as gonorrhea or chlamydia, nor for a diagnosis of AIDS).

Bartholow and colleagues (1994) suggest the lack of research into sexual victimization of gay men is related to the broader lack of awareness and attention to male victims, who have often failed to be recognized as sexually abused. Most of the research has until recently emphasized women as the primary victims of sexual abuse.

To be fair, however, when men are asked about sexual abuse, they report it in far fewer numbers than women do (Becker-Lausen, 1991/1992). In recent years, well-publicized cases of abuse by priests and other male authority figures have raised awareness of the difficulties of reporting for males, which include not only the shame and self-blame generally associated with sexual abuse, but also the compounding factors of a perpetrator's standing in the community and the victim's belief that, as a male, he should have been capable of protecting himself. This latter factor, involving male socialization issues of self-reliance and toughness, makes it particularly difficult to obtain accurate assessments of the range of the problem of male victimization (Finkelhor, 1984; Holmes, Offen & Waller, 1997). This may be even more problematic for victims of abuse by family members than for those abused outside the home. For example, abuse of males by female perpetrators, including caretakers, is an area where there is little empirical documentation (Cermak & Molidor, 1996; Lisak, 1994; Peluso & Putnam, 1996).

For gay men, then, unaddressed issues of traumatic victimization may affect their sexual behavior and their ability to change unsafe practices. Traumatic histories may include sexual abuse, but also may result from verbal and physical abuse related to their status as gay men in a homophobic society. In addition, research into familial sexual abuse within a general population has indicated that it tends to cooccur with other forms of abuse, so that researchers have increasingly argued for a broader definition of child maltreatment which takes this overlap into account (Becker-Lausen & Mallon-Kraft, 1997; Finkelhor & Dziuba-Leatherman, 1994; Sanders & Becker-Lausen, 1995). Future research should further explore these issues in the gay community, so that interventions may be designed that take into account the degree to which all forms of interpersonal trauma may be experienced by an individual within this community.

Alcohol and Other Drugs

Chemically dependent gay men may be particularly in need of treatment for traumatic experiences of childhood, including sexual abuse. Increased rates of child maltreatment have been documented in chemically dependent populations; conversely, survivors of maltreatment are more likely than those without a maltreatment history to have problems with alcohol and other drugs (Briere, 1992). A few studies have documented this relationship for gay men as well (Bartholow et al., 1994; Dimock, 1988); however, these studies have primarily been limited to sexual abuse histories, rather than the broader forms of maltreatment that have been studied in the general population.

For example, Neisen and Sandall (1990) reviewed charts of 201 inpatient lesbians and gay men, age 20 to 39, in treatment for chemical dependency. Nearly 50 percent had chart records indicating they had been sexually abused in childhood. The authors suggest treatment programs must begin to recognize and address these victimization issues in their clients.

In one of the few studies to examine broader child maltreatment issues, 100 gay men in a drug-treatment program were interviewed and completed questionnaires related to familial factors in high-risk sexual behaviors and injection drug use (Neisen, 1993). The study included questions about childhood sexual abuse and other early experiences. However, in the final analyses, the primary predictors of both injection drug use and high-risk sexual behavior were (1) divorce or separation of parents, and (2) parental substance abuse. These findings highlight not only the broader range of experiences that may be traumatic for the child, but also the need for early interventions with high-risk families to prevent the long-term negative outcomes leading to drugs, risky sexual practices, and STDs (Rickel & Becker, 1997).

Cross-training may be needed for mental health professionals working in these areas. Chemical dependency counselors may need to be educated in trauma work and in the specific needs of gay and lesbian clients (Shernoff & Finnegan, 1991). For example, Campbell and Carlson (1995) found a notable lack of appropriate training and knowledge among 427 professionals working with child sexual abuse victims and perpetrators. Less than 40 percent of professionals working with a diverse group of clients, including gay or lesbian perpetrators and victims and culturally diverse individuals, had specific training to work with these populations.

Risk Behavior and Substance Use

Studies of gay and bisexual men have, in general, shown a relationship between substance use and risky sexual behaviors, including unprotected sex and multiple partners (Leigh, 1990; Mulry, Kalichman, & Kelly, 1994; Winters, Remafedi, & Chan, 1996). However, in contrast to these studies in the United States, one study in Great Britain found no relationship between unsafe sex and alcohol use (Weatherburn et al., 1993). Interviews with 461 gay and bisexual men in England and Wales revealed that high-risk sexual behaviors were no more likely to occur when alcohol was used than when it was not. Quantity of alcohol consumed also did not appear to affect sexual risk-taking.

A subsequent report by Perry and colleagues (1994) indicated that alcohol consumption, like other factors related to high-risk behavior, may be a problem only for a subset of gay men. An anonymous survey of 1519 men in gay bars in 16 cities revealed that men who had unprotected anal intercourse after alcohol use were heavier drinkers and engaged in unprotected anal intercourse more frequently than men who had such intercourse when they were not drinking. That is, heavy drinkers were also likely to engage in more high-risk sexual behavior. The Meyer and Dean (1995) study, described earlier in this chapter, appears to confirm this finding of an extremely high-risk subset of individuals. However, for the rest of the sample in the Perry et al. (1994) study, there appeared to be no link between risky sexual behavior and drinking; in general, there was actually *less* unprotected anal intercourse after drinking than without alcohol use.

Some studies have suggested that alcohol and drug use among gay men and lesbians is substantially higher than for the general population (Skinner, 1994), with some estimates as high as one out of every three gay men and lesbians abusing alcohol and drugs (Paul, Stall, & Bloomfield, 1991). However, recent reviews of the research have cited methodological flaws which led to overestimates of the problem (Bux, 1996), and current research has also begun to document declining rates of use among gay men and, to some degree, among lesbians as well, since the beginning of the AIDS epidemic (Paul et al., 1991; Remien et al., 1995).

For gay men participating in a five-year study in the late 1980s and early 1990s, retrospective and prospective data showed significant decreases in use of alcohol and other drugs, and in problems related to substance use (Remien et al., 1995). According to these 56 community subjects, who volunteered to take part in interviews twice a year for the five-year period, the changes in their substance use were related to fear of AIDS and other health issues, decreasing risk-taking behaviors as a means of caring for oneself, and concerns for their self-images.

Abuse of Alcohol and Other Drugs

For specific vulnerable subgroups, however, chemical dependency is a major concern. In a study of 191 gay youth and 75 lesbian youth in two substance abuse treatment programs, most used multiple substances, with alcohol and marijuana the most common mix (Shifrin & Solis, 1992). Furthermore, abuse of alcohol and other drugs has been identified across numerous studies as a consistent predictor of high-risk sexual behavior for all groups at risk for HIV infection, including gay and bisexual men, injection drug users, and also heterosexual youth and adults (Kalichman, Kelly, & St. Lawrence, 1990).

In one study of 314 gay and bisexual men from San Francisco in substance abuse treatment, a control group was developed from the San Francisco Men's Health Study, a prospective investigation of AIDS risk in single men (Paul et al., 1993). The control group consisted of 586 self-identified gay or bisexual men. When the substance abuse group was compared to the health study control sample, sexual risk behaviors were significantly higher among the substance-abusing men than among the community sample. Among subjects in outpatient treatment for substance abuse, 23 percent reported unprotected receptive anal sex, compared to 15 percent of controls; 21 percent reported unprotected insertive anal sex, compared to 17 percent of the control group. In the prior three months, 32 percent of the substance abusers reported unprotected anal sex (insertive and/or receptive), whereas 22 percent of the community subjects reported engaging in these behaviors during a previous six-month period.

Focus groups with the substance abuse subjects revealed issues subjects perceived as limiting their ability to change risky behavior (Paul et al., 1993). These issues included perceptions of the disinhibiting effects of alcohol and other drugs, established associations of substance use with sex, as well as personality factors such as low self-esteem, lack of assertiveness, lack of skills for negotiating with partners, and a sense of powerlessness. The authors note that few prevention strategies have been developed that specifically target substance-abusing gay men. Yet techniques used in substance abuse treatment, such as relapse·prevention and motivational interviewing (Rickel & Becker-Lausen, 1994), have useful applications in the prevention of high-risk sexual behavior as well (Miller & Rollnick, 1991), and thus could be readily incorporated into treatment programs for gay men.

Personality Factors

Regarding personality factors associated with high-risk behavior, subsequent empirical studies have supported and further delineated the qualitative findings from focus groups identified in the study by Paul and colleagues (1993). Among 416 gay men attending a clinic for STDs, a significant relationship was identified between proactive coping strategies (i.e., problem-focused strategies, such as seeking advice or support) and lower rates of drug use, fewer sexual partners, and less frequent sexual activity (Barrett et al., 1995). Strategies categorized as emotion-focused coping, such as denial and distancing in relationships, were significantly related to use of more types of drugs. Engaging in high-risk sexual behavior (such as unprotected anal intercourse) was less consistently related to problem-focused coping styles (with the exception of support-seeking). Unprotected anal intercourse was also more consistently related to an emotion-focused coping style.

Partner Intimidation, Coercion, and Violence

Gay men and lesbian women are often victims of antigay violence from the larger community. In one sample of gay and lesbian college students documenting antigay harassment and discrimination (D'Augelli, 1992a), 77 percent of subjects had been verbally insulted, 27 percent had been threatened with physical violence, 13 percent experienced property damage, 22 percent had been chased, and 5 percent had been physically assaulted. Few of these students reported these incidents, which were primarily initiated by fellow students. Other studies have found similar results with adolescents (Hunter, 1990) and with college students (Herek, 1993).

Few studies have investigated the prevalence of coercion and violence within the gay community, however. Baier, Rosenzweig, and Whipple (1991) investigated the extent of sexual coercion within a university sample of 340 male and 362 female students. Coercion and victimization rates were analyzed by gender, class level, and sexual orientation. More than one-third of gay/bisexual subjects indicated they had engaged in sexual intercourse under what they experienced as coercion, when they did not want to have sex. One-fourth of the women subjects reported this experience, and one-eighth of male subjects said they had experienced it. More than 50 percent of these experiences occurred before subjects entered college.

To examine the relationship between sexual coercion and high-risk sexual behavior, Kalichman and Rompa (1995) assessed the sexual behavior of 196 gay and bisexual men for a three-month period prior to their study. Similar to the findings for college students, 29 percent of these gay/bisexual subjects reported they had been coerced into sexual contact when they did not want it. Significantly, 92 percent of these encounters involved unprotected anal intercourse, supporting the premise that sexual coercion may be a major factor in risky sexual practices. Intention to reduce risky behaviors was reported both by subjects who reported coercion and those who did not; however, subjects who felt coerced anticipated less engagement in behaviors to resist risky practices in the future. Thus, skills training in risk-reduction strategies may be an important element to be included in prevention efforts with this population.

Like child maltreatment, the issue of violence between partners and its effects on sexual behavior has not been adequately studied in the gay community. Future research needs to explore and identify factors that are specific to the needs of this population. For example, the problems of prejudice and antigay violence may make the discussion of partner violence more difficult. Studies indicate that gay and lesbian battering is underreported and unlikely to be disclosed by the victim (American Psychological Association, 1996). The problem appears to be similar to that of African-American women, who may hesitate to report battering by African-American men, because of legitimate concerns about injustice and unequal treatment by law enforcement. Both quantitative and qualitative studies are needed to determine the most appropriate intervention for this community, one that would be sensitive to all of these issues.

ISSUES IN TREATMENT

Living with AIDS

In the 1990s, the major breakthrough for AIDS patients has been the success of new drug therapies that have begun to turn the disease from a death sentence into a chronic illness (Beaudin & Chambre, 1996). These changes have required new medical and psychological approaches which address medical, social, and epidemiological factors of chronicity, rather than crisis management.

From the perspective of the practitioner working with AIDS patients, this shift may have dramatic effects on their clients' perspectives, as described by Barret (1997, Summer):

A client who had sold his business and distributed most of his estate to relatives is absorbed in seeking ways to reclaim the capital that might enable him to start another business. Another has initiated a serious conversation with his lover, suddenly aware that the relationship he might tolerate as long as he was sick is simply unacceptable now that he is feeling better. One 30-year-old who had come home to die but never got sick, was astounded with a sudden realization while driving his delivery truck. "I'm not going to die. I am going to live. Suddenly I have a chance to have a life, something that I thought was over for me." (p. 1)

Interviews with 55 HIV-positive gay men, age 22 to 53 years, revealed the primary tasks of adaptation to the disease, which suggest it has aspects of other chronic ailments, but also its own unique elements (Siegel & Krauss, 1991). Beyond a continued concern with the possibility of a shortened life, the men in this study were facing the challenge of others' reactions to the stigma of the disease, and the task of developing ways to enhance and maintain both their physical and emotional health.

Kalichman (1995) delineated some of the salient themes which recur in psychotherapy with HIV-positive clients. These include changing behavior and lifestyle to promote better health, issues of disclosure of status (both to loved ones and to others), effects of the diagnosis on the client's relationships, problems with substance abuse, considerations of suicide, making meaningful use of time, and spirituality.

Partners of AIDS Patients

Partners of AIDS patients may need specialized services themselves. Studies of caregiving partners have revealed they suffer psychologically and even physically from the strain of caregiving, but especially from bereavement at the partner's death.

In this arena, as in risk-prevention, coping skills make a difference. Interviews with 37 HIV-positive and 73 HIV-negative caregiving partners, aged 24 to 57, indicated subjects used more problem-focused coping strategies (such as those described above for risky sex and substance abuse) during caregiving than during bereavement (Moskowitz, Folkman, Collette, & Vittinghoff, 1996). Cognitive escape avoidance was also more common during caregiving periods than after death. Negative and positive moods were associated with different coping styles, but the caregivers' own HIV status had no effect on the mood and coping relationship.

In another analysis of the same group of interviews, Folkman and colleagues (Folkman, Chesney, Collette, Boccellari, & Cooke, 1996) examined the depression scores of these caregivers three months before and seven months after their partners' deaths. During the entire 10-month period, caregivers' average scores were clinically elevated, indicating they were at risk for a major depressive episode. In the seven months after the partner's death, depression scores decreased in 63 percent of the sample, but the remaining 37 percent showed continued high scores. Decreasing depression after the partner's death was associated with higher depression scores before the death and with the ability to find positive meaning in the caregiving experience. Continued high scores for depression were predicted by HIV-positive status of the caregiver, longer term relationships with the partner, experiencing hassles in the environment, and the use of self-blaming and distancing as coping mechanisms.

In another study (Kemeny et al., 1995), decreases in immune function were documented in 39 HIV-positive men following the death of an intimate partner from AIDS. The immune changes seen were ones that could negatively affect the progression of AIDS.

Traumatic Stress, Grief, and Loss in the Gay Community

Although it has been predicted that the multiple losses to AIDS experienced by members of the gay community constitute a significant traumatic experience that would complicate bereavement for most individuals involved (Nord, 1996), studies have not consistently supported this proposition.

In a study of 93 gay men in San Francisco who had lost at least three friends, relatives, or lovers to AIDS (and who were either HIV negative or did not know their status), no significant relationship was found between number of losses and the intensity of the grief experience (Cherney & Verhey, 1996).

More specifically, researchers in Australia predicted that gay males in two communities experiencing differing levels of loss would show differences in anxiety, depression, and anger (Viney, Henry, Walker, & Crooks, 1992). Among the 215 gay males, aged 23 to 55, in the two communities, those from the more bereaved group did, in fact, report higher levels of anxiety and anger, but the two communities did not differ in regard to their rates of depression.

Other studies have indicated that the individual's own HIV status may be a factor in bereavement effects (Martin & Dean, 1993), as well as the individual's role as a caregiver to a dying AIDS patient and the adequacy of their social support systems (Lennon, Martin, & Dean, 1990).

Finally, there is limited evidence from research that sexual behavior may be affected by fear and grief associated with AIDS losses (Ames, Atchinson, & Rose, 1995). In a study of 280 gay men in small cities, AIDS was found to be a factor that was continually within the men's awareness, although not necessarily ruling their lives. Those who use condoms consistently report fear as a primary factor in their behavior, yet most subjects say they are attempting to balance protection with sexual satisfaction and with the need for intimate bonding with others. Continued risk-taking was found in this community, despite these responses. Researchers emphasize the need for continued intervention within the gay community which takes into account all of these psychosocial factors of decision-making.

GUIDELINES FOR INTERVENTION

Based on the studies conducted within the gay community and reviewed in this chapter, the following guidelines are proposed.

Strategies Most Likely to Succeed

As a group, gay men have shown a great deal of facility for changing their high-risk sexual behavior. However, individual differences appear to be significant factors affecting long-term changes. As with other populations, higher levels of informal social support and active seeking of social support are good predictors of who is able to change and likely to maintain safe sex practices. In addition, as with other groups, a sense of self-efficacy, particularly the expectation that safe sex has positive personal and interpersonal outcomes, is associated with changing behavior and maintaining changes. Negative expectations about the difficulties of safer sex, faulty beliefs about risk, and a belief that the individual had little personal control over prevention of AIDS were associated with high-risk behavior and with difficulty sustaining positive changes in behavior. Thus, the prevention models described in Chapter 3, which include increasing knowledge, enhancing social support and peer acceptance of safer sex practices, building a sense of mastery, and stressing the positive aspects of safer sex, are important in working within the gay community. Stressing the need for safe sex practices even in longer-term relationships is also important, although it may be among the most difficult concepts for groups to accept. Issues of partner coercion and/or violence must be addressed more openly in the gay community, given the relationship that has been documented between coercion and high-risk sexual behavior.

Younger gay and bisexual men and ethnic minority gay and bisexual men appear to be at significantly greater risk than their older, white counterparts; interventions must be designed using peers and role models who are similar in characteristics or who are part of these at-risk groups. Outreach campaigns must be designed to go directly into the community with one-on-one interventions, particularly where poverty levels are high, educational levels are low, and drug use is prevalent.

Institutionalized maltreatment, whether in the form of racism or homophobia, hits gay and bisexual youth and minority members the hardest. In addition, where other forms of maltreatment are also present in the individual's life, such as the deprivation associated with poverty, the effects of street violence and of family violence (including child abuse and neglect), parental substance abuse or divorce, or the effects of extrafamilial sexual abuse, the individual may be severely traumatized and less able to benefit from standard interventions.

Attention to these individual risk elements, particularly psychological factors associated with trauma history, may require considerably more attention to individually tailored interventions for the highest risk members of the community. Given the findings that a small subset of the gay community engages in the highest risk behaviors, these individualized plans may be critical in decreasing risk for the community at large. Designing these interventions for use with patients at clinics for STDs, given the relationship between STDs and HIV infection, may be one place to begin to reach these high-risk individuals. Motivational interviewing techniques should be part of the armamentarium of all health workers delivering direct services in these clinics.

Substance abuse treatment programs are also critical points of entry for intervention around safer sex practices. Clinicians working with substance abusers should be thoroughly trained in working with the effects of trauma, as well as in work with diverse populations, particularly gay or bisexual men, lesbian or bisexual women, and ethnic minority clients. Mental health clinicians who work primarily with trauma also need to be aware of the opportunity to address high-risk sexual practices and substance abuse risk, and to be trained in work with a diversity of sexual orientations and ethnic groups. All health care providers need to be well trained in the issue of partner coercion and violence, including knowing how to ask questions and understanding the specific sensitivities of culturally diverse groups, particularly those who have reason to fear discrimination and prejudicial attitudes from police or other authories.

High-risk groups also include gay and bisexual men in nonurban communities, where again the younger and less educated men are the most at risk. Bisexual men may respond to interventions aimed at their lifestyle, using bisexual peers and role models to change normative expectations, provide education regarding the positive aspects of prevention, increase motivation, and teach behavioral skills.

Special attention also must be paid to the needs of HIV-positive gay men and their caregiving partners. In addition to individual psychotherapy where grief and loss issues may be addressed (both before and after death), research again suggests that enhancing social support systems, increasing motivation to engage in healthier behaviors, and building the individual's sense of self-efficacy around prevention skills remain important aspects of intervention.

Ineffective Strategies

Educational campaigns, including the use of mass media techniques, are unlikely to effectively reach the most vulnerable members of the gay population. Traditional intervention campaigns have been fairly effective with white, adult, educated gay men, but have generally failed to reach ethnic minority men, younger men, and bisexual men in the community.

Epilogue

What can we conclude about prevention of high-risk sexual behavior? First, we still have much to learn about effective prevention, particularly with regard to issues of cultural diversity. We also need a better understanding of the relationship between preventing teen pregnancy and preventing STDs, including AIDS.

The cost of our failure to prevent these consequences should be abundantly clear, including tremendous human suffering, health care costs, loss of productivity, illness, death, child maltreatment, welfare dependency, and multigenerational poverty.

In addition to these outcomes, we have described how high-risk sexual behavior is inextricably linked to other societal problems, including substance abuse, violence and victimization, homelessness, and poverty.

Research efforts so far have provided prevention strategies with a strong probability of success. A combination of increasing knowledge, enhancing motivation, and building competencies appears to have the best chance of effectively changing sexual risk behavior. Programs using these techniques are being implemented and further tested by researchers. Assessing stages of change also seems to be a useful technique for effective intervention, and the earlier the intervention in a youth's life, the better chance it has of succeeding. As with prevention of other sexual risk outcomes, multiple levels of intervention may be necessary to prevent teen pregnancy and to prevent a second pregnancy with the adolescent mother. Parenting teens are helped most by longer term programs (a minimum of seven weeks).

Regarding ethnicity factors, more research is needed to design and assess prevention efforts with specific ethnic groups. Notably lacking is research with Asian Americans and with Native Americans. Work so far with diverse groups has indicated that the combination of increasing knowledge, enhancing motivation, and building competencies works well across cultural groups; however, these efforts appear to be more effective when materials, role models, and presenters are culturally appropriate. Furthermore, poverty is a factor that must be addressed effectively before efforts at prevention are likely to succeed on any large scale.

Similar findings have been reported for women. Poverty is a major factor that must be addressed simultaneously, or sexual risk prevention is unlikely to have widespread success. For women, issues of violence and sexual coercion are also important factors. Again, the knowledge, motivation, and competency model is effective; for women the building of skills in introducing safe sex practices is particularly important.

Efforts within the gay community have been relatively successful in recent years; however, there are signs these gains are at risk of being lost. Younger gay and bisexual men, ethnic minority gay and bisexual men, poorer and less educated gay and bisexual men, as well as those who have experienced child maltreatment, who are addicted to alcohol or other drugs, and who live in nonurban communities are especially in need of targeted intervention programs that are sensitive to their needs. Grief and loss issues must also be addressed within the gay community.

For all of these groups, in addition to the triad of knowledge, motivation, and competency-building, social support systems are also key to effective prevention. Therefore, enhancing our communities, so that support structures emerge for all individuals within the community, will do a great deal to move us toward a world where no one is left out, where individuals find the energy and will to prevent negative consequences and to build a better life for themselves and for their loved ones.

References

Abel, E. L. (Ed.). (1996). *Fetal alcohol syndrome: From mechanism to prevention.* Boca Raton, FL: CRC Press.

Adler, N. (1992). Unwanted pregnancy and abortion: Definitional and research issues. *Journal of Social Issues, 48* (3), 19–35.

Adler, N. (1994). *Adolescent sexual behavior looks irrational—But looks are deceiving.* Science and Public Policy Seminars. Washington, DC: Federation of Behavioral, Psychological, and Cognitive Sciences.

Adler, N., David, H., Major, B., Roth, S., Russo, N., & Wyatt, G. (1990). Psychological responses after abortion. *Science, 248,* 41–44.

Alan Guttmacher Institute. (1986). *Teenage pregnancy in industrialized countries: A study.* New Haven: Yale University Press.

Alan Guttmacher Institute. (1994). *Teenage reproductive health in the United States.* New York: Author.

Alan Guttmacher Institute. (1995, February). Teen pregnancy and the welfare reform debate. *Issues in Brief,* 1–4.

Alexander, N. J. (1996). Sexual spread of HIV infection. *Human Reproduction, 11* (7 Supplement), 111–120.

American College Health Association. (1990). *Making sex safer.* (Brochure). Baltimore, MD: Author.

American Psychiatric Association. (1994). *Diagnostic and statistical manual of mental disorders* (4th ed.). Washington, DC: Author.

American Psychological Association. (1996). *Violence and the family. Report of the American Psychological Association Presidential Task Force on Violence and the Family.* Washington, DC: Author.

Ames, L. J., Atchinson, A. B., & Rose, D. T. (1995). Love, lust, and fear: Safer sex decision making among gay men. *Journal of Homosexuality, 30* (1), 53–73.

Anderson, R. N., Kochanek, K. D., & Murphy, S. L. (1997). Report of final mortality statistics, 1995. *Monthly Vital Statistics Report, 45* (11, Supplement 2), National Center for Health Statistics.

Ankrah, E. M. (1995). Let their voices be heard: Empowering women in the fight against AIDS. *AIDS Captions, 2* (3), 4–7.

Azjen, I., & Fishbein, M. (1980). *Understanding attitudes and predicting social behavior.* Englewood Cliffs, NJ: Prentice-Hall.

Bagley, C., & Young, L. (1987). Juvenile prostitution and child sexual abuse: A controlled study. *Canadian Journal of Community Mental Health, 6* (1), 5–26.

Baier, J. L., Rosenzweig, M. G., & Whipple, E. G. (1991). Patterns of sexual behavior, coercion, and victimization of university students. *Journal of College Student Development, 32,* 310–322.

Bandura, A. (1986). *The social foundations of thought and action.* Englewood Cliffs, NJ: Prentice-Hall.

Barret, B. (1997, Summer). Life on the edge: Cherishing the lessons, holding on to the hope. *Psychology and AIDS Exchange,* Issue 23. Washington, DC: American Psychological Association.

Barrett, D. C., Bolan, G., Joy, D., Counts, K., Doll, L., & Harrison, J. (1995). Coping strategies, substance use, sexual activity, and HIV sexual risks in a sample of gay male STD patients. *Journal of Applied Social Psychology, 25,* 1058–1072.

Bartholow, B. N., Doll, L. S., Joy, D., Douglas, J. M., Jr., Bolan, G., Harrison, J. S., Moss, P. M., & McKirnan, D. (1994). Emotional, behavioral, and HIV risks associated with sexual abuse among adult homosexual and bisexual men. *Child Abuse and Neglect, 18,* 747–761.

Beaudin, C. L., & Chambre, S. M. (1996). HIV/AIDS as a chronic disease: Emergence from the plague model. *American Behavioral Scientist, 39,* 684–706.

Beck, A. T. (1972). *Depression: Causes and treatment.* Philadelphia: University of Pennsylvania Press.

Beck, J. G., & Davies, D. K. (1987). Teen contraception: A review of perspectives on compliance. *Archives of Sexual Behavior, 16,* 337–368.

Becker, J. V., Skinner, L. J., Abel, G. G., & Chichon, J. (1986). Level of post-assault sexual functioning in rape and incest victims. *Archives of Sexual Behavior, 15,* 37–49.

Becker-Lausen, E. (1992). Child abuse and negative life experiences: An analysis of depression and dissociation as mediator variables. (Doctoral dissertation, University of Connecticut, 1991). *Dissertation Abstracts International, 53* (1B), 557.

Becker-Lausen, E., & Gleeson, M. K. (1996, May). *Child maltreatment and high-risk sexual behavior: Data from two diverse populations.* Paper presented at the 73rd Annual Meeting of the American Orthopsychiatric Association, Boston, MA.

Becker-Lausen, E., and Mallon-Kraft, S. (1997). Pandemic outcomes: The intimacy variable. In G. Kaufman Kantor & J. Jasinski (Eds.), *Out of darkness: Contemporary research perspectives on family violence* (pp. 49–57). Thousand Oaks, CA: Sage.

Becker-Lausen, E., & Rickel, A. U. (1995). Integration of teen pregnancy and child abuse research: Identifying mediator variables for pregnancy outcome. *The Journal of Primary Prevention, 16,* 39–53.

Becker-Lausen, E., Sanders, B., & Chinsky, J. M. (1995). Mediation of abusive childhood experiences: Depression, dissociation, and negative life outcomes. *American Journal of Orthopsychiatry, 65* (4), 560–573.

Belongia, E. A., Danila, R. N., Angamuthu, V., Hickman, C. D., DeBoer, J. M., MacDonald, K. L., & Osterholm, M. T. (1997). A population-based study of sexually transmitted disease incidence and risk factors in human immunodeficiency virus-infected people. *Sexually Transmitted Diseases, 24,* 251–256.

Bernstein, E. M., & Putnam, F. W. (1986). Development, reliability, and validity of a dissociation scale. *Journal of Nervous and Mental Disease, 174,* 727–735.

Biglan, A. (1993). Recapturing Skinner's legacy to behavior therapy. *Behavior Therapist, 16,* 3–5.

Biglan, A., Metzler, C. W., Wirt, R., Ary, D., Noell, J., Ochs, L., French, C., & Hood, D. (1990). Social and behavioral factors associated with high-risk sexual behavior among adolescents. *Journal of Behavioral Medicine, 13,* 245–261.

Biglan, A., Noell, J., Ochs, L., Smolkowski, K., & Metzler, C. (1995). Does sexual coercion play a role in the high-risk sexual behavior of adolescent and young adult women? *Journal of Behavioral Medicine, 18*, 549–568.

Billy, J., Tanfer, K., Grady, W., & Klepinger, D. (1993). The sexual behavior of men in the United States. *Family Planning Perspectives, 25*, 52–60.

Block, J. (1965). *The Child Rearing Practices Report*. Berkeley: University of California, Institute of Human Development.

Bochow, M., Chiarotti, F., Davies, P., Dubois-Arber, F., Dur, W., Fouchard, J., Gruet, F., McManus, T., Markert, S., Sandfort, T., Sasse, H., Schiltz, M. A., Tielman, R., & Wasserfallen, F. (1994). Sexual behavior of gay and bisexual men in eight European countries. *AIDS Care, 6*, 533–549.

Botvin, G. J., Schinke, S., & Orlandi, M. A. (1995). School-based health promotion: Substance abuse and sexual behavior. *Applied and Preventive Psychology, 4*, 167–184.

Bownes, I. T., O'Gorman, E. C., & Sayers, A. (1991). Psychiatric symptoms, behavioural responses and post-traumatic stress disorder in rape victims. *Issues in Criminological and Legal Psychology, 1* (17), 25–33.

Bowser, B. P., Fullilove, M. T., & Fullilove, R. E. (1990). African-American youth and high-risk AIDS behavior: The social context and barriers to prevention. *Youth & Society, 22* (1), 54–66.

Boyer, D., & Fine, D. (1989, November). *Sexual abuse as a factor in adolescent pregnancy and child maltreatment: Preliminary data from a longitudinal study*. Paper presented at the Fall Grantees Meeting of the National Center on Abuse and Neglect, Washington, DC.

Braverman, P. K., & Strasburger, V. C. (1993). Adolescent sexuality: Part 2. Contraception. *Clinical Pediatrics, 32*, 725–734.

Briere, J. N. (1992). *Child abuse trauma: Theory and treatment of the lasting effects*. Newbury Park, CA: Sage.

Briere, J. N., & Runtz, M. (1988). Symptomology associated with child sexual victimization in a nonclinical adult sample. *Child Abuse and Neglect, 12*, 51–59.

Brown, W. J. (1992). Culture and AIDS education: Reaching high-risk heterosexuals in Asian-American communities. *Journal of Applied Communication Research, 20* (3), 275–291.

Browne, A., & Finkelhor, D. (1986). Impact of child sexual abuse: A review of the research. *Psychological Bulletin, 99* (1), 66–77.

Bux, D. A., Jr. (1996). The epidemiology of problem drinking in gay men and lesbians: A critical review. *Clinical Psychology Review, 16*, 277–298.

Calhoun, K. S., & Resick, P. A. (1993). Post-traumatic stress disorder. In D. H. Barlow (Ed.), *Clinical handbook of psychological disorders: A step-by-step treatment manual* (2nd ed., pp. 48–98). New York: Guilford.

Campbell, J. A., & Carlson, K. (1995). Training and knowledge of professionals on specific topics in child sexual abuse. *Journal of Child Sexual Abuse, 4* (1), 75–86.

Carey, R. F., Herman, W. A., Retta, S. M., Rinaldi, J. E., Herman, B. A., & Athey, T. W. (1992). Effectiveness of latex condoms as a barrier to human immunodeficiency virus-sized particles under conditions of simulated use. *Sexually Transmitted Diseases, 19*, 230–234.

Carson, S. (1997). Human papillomatous virus infection update: Impact on women's health. *Nurse Practitioner: American Journal of Primary Health Care, 22* (4), 24–25, 28, 30.

Cassiday, K. L., McNally, R. J., & Zeitlin, S. B. (1992). Cognitive processing of trauma cues in rape victims with post-traumatic stress disorder. *Cognitive Therapy and Research, 16*, 283–295.

Catania, J., Coates, T., Greenblatt, R., Dolcini, M., Kegeles, S., Puckett, S., Corman, M., & Miller, J. (1989). Predictors of condom use and multiple partnered sex among sexually active adolescent women: Implications for AIDS-related health interventions. *Journal of Sex Research, 26*, 514–524.

Catania, J., Coates, T., Stall, R., Bye, L., Kegeles, S., Capell, F., Henne, J., McKusick, L., Morin, S., & Turner, H. (1991). Changes in condom use among homosexual men in San Francisco. *Health Psychology, 10* (3), 190–199.

Centers for Disease Control (1992, April). *HIV/AIDS surveillance report*. Atlanta: Author.

Centers for Disease Control. (1993, July). *HIV/AIDS surveillance report*. Atlanta: Author.

Centers for Disease Control (1994a). Heterosexually acquired AIDS: United States, 1993. *Morbidity and Mortality Weekly Report, 43*, 155–160.

Centers for Disease Control (1994b). U. S. AIDS cases reported through December 1993. *HIV/AIDS surveillance report*. Atlanta: Author.

Centers for Disease Control (1995). *HIV/AIDS surveillance report*. Atlanta: Author.

Centers for Disease Control (1996a). AIDS associated with injecting-drug use: United States, 1995. *Morbidity and Mortality Weekly Report, 45*, 392–398.

Centers for Disease Control (1996b). *HIV/AIDS surveillance report*. Atlanta: Author.

Centers for Disease Control and Prevention, HIV/AIDS Prevention Program (1997, September). www.cdc.gov/nchstp/hiv_aids/graphics/women.htm

Cermak, P., & Molidor, C. (1996). Male victims of child sexual abuse. *Child and Adolescent Social Work Journal, 13*, 385–400.

Cherney, P. M., & Verhey, M. P. (1996). Grief among gay men associated with multiple losses from AIDS. *Death Studies, 20*, 115–132.

Choi, K. H., & Coates, T. J. (1994). Prevention of HIV infection. *AIDS, 8*, 1371–1389.

Choi, K. H., Coates, T. J., Catania, J. A., Lew, S., & Chow, P. (1995). High HIV risk among gay Asian and Pacific Islander men in San Francisco. *AIDS, 9*, 306–307.

Cleavenger, R. L., Juckett, R. G., & Hobbs, G. R. (1996). Trends in chlamydia and other sexually transmitted diseases in a university health service. *Journal of American College Health, 44*, 263–265.

Cline, R. J. W. (1991). *Dangerous liaisons: Challenging the assumptions of interpersonal AIDS-prevention advice*. Paper presented at the International Communication Association, Chicago, IL.

Cline, R. J. W., & McKenzie, N. J. (1994). Sex differences in communication and the construction of HIV/AIDS. *Journal of Applied Communication Research, 22*, 322–337.

Coates, T. J. (1990). Strategies for modifying sexual behavior for primary and secondary prevention of HIV disease. *Journal of Consulting and Clinical Psychology, 58* (1), 57–69.

Cochran, S. D., de Leeuw, J., & Mays, V. M. (1995). Optimal scaling of HIV-related sexual risk behaviors in ethnically diverse homosexually active men. *Journal of Consulting and Clinical Psychology, 63*, 270–279.

Cole, F. L., & Slocumb, E. M. (1995). Factors influencing safer sexual behaviors in heterosexual late adolescent and young adult collegiate males. *Image: Journal of Nursing Scholarship, 27*, 217–223.

Conger, R. D., Ge, X., Elder, G. H., Jr., Lorenz, F. O., & Simons, R. L. (1994). Economic stress, coercive family process, and developmental problems of adolescents. *Child Development, 65*, 541–561.

Conner, J. L., & Conner, C. N. (1992). Expected benefits of alcohol use on sexual behavior: Native American adolescents. *Psychological Reports, 70*, 91–98.

Croteau, J. M., Nero, C. I., & Prosser, D. J. (1993). Social and cultural sensitivity in group-specific HIV and AIDS programming. *Journal of Counseling and Development, 71*, 290–296.

Cummings, M., & Cummings, S. (1983). Family planning among the urban poor: Sexual politics and social policy. *Family Relations Journal of Applied Family and Child Studies, 32* (1), 47–58.

Curtin, L., Stephens, R. S., & Roffman, R. A. (1997). Determinants of relapse and the rule violation effect in predicting safer sex goal violations. *Journal of Applied Social Psychology, 27*, 649–663.

Dabrow, S. M., Merrick, C. L., & Conlon, M. (1995). Adolescent girls' attitudes toward contraceptive subdermal implants. *Journal of Adolescent Health, 16,* 360–366.

Damond, M. E., Breuer, N. L., & Pharr, A. E. (1993). The evaluation of setting and a culturally specific HIV/AIDS curriculum: HIV/AIDS knowledge and behavioral intent of African American adolescents. *Journal of Black Psychology, 19* (2), 169–189.

D'Augelli, A. R. (1992a). Lesbian and gay male undergraduates' experiences of harassment and fear on campus. *Journal of Interpersonal Violence, 7,* 383–395.

D'Augelli, A. R. (1992b). Sexual behavior patterns of gay university men: Implications for preventing HIV infection. *Journal of American College Health, 41* (1), 25–29.

Davidson, J. K., & Moore, N. B. (1994). Guilt and lack of orgasm during sexual intercourse: Myth versus reality among college women. *Journal of Sex Education and Therapy, 20* (3), 153–174.

Davidson, J. R., Hughes, D., Blazer, D. G., & George, L. K. (1991). Post-traumatic stress disorder in the community: An epidemiological study. *Psychological Medicine, 21,* 713–721.

Davies, K. (1990). Genital herpes: An overview. *Journal of Obstetric, Gynecologic and Neonatal Nursing, 19,* 401–406.

Davis, S. M., & Harris, M. B. (1982). Sexual knowledge, sexual interests, and sources of sexual information of rural and urban adolescents from three cultures. *Adolescence, 17,* 471–492.

Dawson, J. M., Fitzpatrick, R. M., Reeves, G., Boulton, M., McLean, J., Hart, G. J., & Brookes, M. (1994). Awareness of sexual partners' HIV status as an influence upon high-risk sexual behaviour among gay men. *AIDS, 8,* 837–841.

Derksen, D. J. (1992). Children with condylomata acuminata. *Journal of Family Practice, 34,* 419–423.

Desmond, A. M. (1994). Adolescent pregnancy in the United States: Not a minority issue. *Health Care for Women International, 15,* 325–331.

deWit, J. B.F., & van Griensvan, G. J.P. (1994). Time from safer to unsafe sexual behaviour among homosexual men. *AIDS, 8,* 123–126.

Dignan, M. B. (1979). Locus of control, perceived susceptibility to pregnancy and choice of contraceptive among college students. *Perceptual and Motor Skills, 48,* 782.

Dignan, M. B., & Adame, D. D. (1979). Locus of control and human sexuality education. *Perceptual and Motor Skills, 49,* 778.

Dimock, P. (1988). Adult males sexually abused as children. *Journal of Interpersonal Violence, 3,* 203–221.

Division of STD Prevention (1997, September). *Sexually transmitted disease surveillance, 1996.* Atlanta: Centers for Disease Control and Prevention, U.S. Public Health Service.

Eby, K. K., Campbell, J. C., Sullivan, C. M., & Davidson, W. S. (1995). Health effects of experiences of sexual violence for women with abusive partners. *Health Care for Women International, 16,* 563–576.

Einhorn, L., & Polgar, M. (1994). HIV-risk behavior among lesbians and bisexual women. *AIDS Education and Prevention, 6,* 514–523.

el Bassel, N., & Schilling, R. F. (1992). 15-month followup of women methadone patients taught skills to reduce heterosexual HIV transmission. *Public Health Reports, 107* (5), 500–504.

Ellis, E. M., Calhoun, K. S., & Atkeson, B. M. (1980). Sexual dysfunctions in victims of rape: Victims may experience a loss of sexual arousal and frightening flashbacks even one year after the assault. *Women and Health, 5,* 39–47.

Emans, S. J., (1983). The sexually active teenager. *Journal of Developmental and Behavioral Pediatrics, 4* (1), 37–42.

Ericksen, K. P., & Trocki, K. F. (1992). Behavioral risk factors for sexually transmitted diseases in American households. *Social Science and Medicine, 34,* 843–853.

Erickson, P., & Rapkin, A. J. (1991). Unwanted sexual experiences among middle and high school youth. *Journal of Adolescent Health, 12,* 319–325.

Erikson, R. C. (1993). Abortion trauma: Application of a conflict model. *Pre- and Peri-Natal Psychology Journal, 8* (1), 33–42.

Evans, J. K., Holmes, A., Browning, M., & Forster, G. E. (1996). Emergency hormonal contraception usage in genitourinary medicine clinic attenders. *Genitourinary Medicine, 72* (3), 217–219.

Exner, T. M., Meyer-Bahlburg, H. F., & Ehrhardt, A. A. (1992). Sexual self control as a mediator of high risk sexual behavior in a New York City cohort of HIV+ and HIV– gay men. *Journal of Sex Research, 29,* 389–406.

Ferreira, N. (1996). Sexually transmitted Chlamydia trachomatis. *Nurse Practitioner Forum, 7,* 40–46.

Finkelhor, D. (1984). Sexual abuse of boys. In A. W. Burgess (Ed.), *Research handbook on rape and sexual assault* (pp. 97–109). New York: Garland

Finkelhor, D., & Dziuba-Leatherman, J. (1994). Victimization of children. *American Psychologist, 49* (3), 173–183.

Fisher, J. D., & Fisher, W. A. (1992). Changing AIDS risk behavior. *Psychological Bulletin, 111,* 455–474.

Fisher, J. D., & Fisher, W. A. (1995, May 1). Changing AIDS risk behavior in high school students. A proposal submitted to NIMH. Unpublished manuscript, University of Connecticut, Storrs.

Fisher, J. D., Fisher, W. A., Williams, S. S., & Malloy, T. E. (1994). Empirical tests of an information-motivation-behavioral skills model of AIDS preventive behavior. *Health Psychology, 13,* 238–250.

Fisher, W. A., & Fisher, J. D. (1993). A general social psychological model for changing AIDS risk behavior. In J. Pryor & G. Reeder (Eds.), *The social psychology of HIV infection* (pp. 127–153). Hillsdale, NJ: Erlbaum.

Flores-Ortiz, Y. G. (1994). The role of cultural and gender values in alcohol use patterns among Chicana/Latina high school and university students: Implications for AIDS prevention. *International Journal of the Addictions, 29,* 1149–1171.

Folkman, S., Chesney, M., Collette, L., Boccellari, A., & Cooke, M. (1996). Postbereavement depressive mood and its prebereavement predictors in HIV+ and HIV– gay men. *Journal of Personality and Social Psychology, 70,* 336–348.

Forgatch, M. S., & Stoolmiller, M. (1994). Emotions as contexts for adolescent delinquency. *Journal of Research on Adolescence, 4,* 601–614.

Freud, S. (1964). Beyond the pleasure principle. In J. Strachey (Ed.), *The standard edition of the complete psychological works of Sigmund Freud* (Vol. 18, pp. 7–64). London: Hogarth Press. (Original work published 1920)

Friedman, H. L. (1989). The health of adolescents: Beliefs and behavior. *Social Science and Medicine, 29,* 309–315.

Fromuth, M. E. (1983, August). The long term psychological impact of childhood sexual abuse. Unpublished doctoral dissertation, Auburn University, Auburn, AL.

Furstenberg, F. F., Jr., Brooks-Gunn, J., & Morgan, S. P. (1987). *Adolescent mothers in later life.* New York: Cambridge University Press.

Garbarino, J. (1995). *Raising children in a socially toxic environment.* San Francisco: Jossey-Bass Publishers.

Gayle, H. D., & D'Angelo, L. J. (1991). Epidemiology of acquired immunodeficiency syndrome and human immunodeficiency virus infection in adolescents. *Pediatric Infectious Disease Journal, 10,* 322–328.

Ghys, P. D., Diallo, M. O., Ettiegne-Traore, V., Yeboue, K. M., Gnaore, E., Lorougnon, F., Teurquetil, M. J., Adom, M. L., Greenberg, A. E., & Laga, M. (1995). Dual seroreactivity to HIV-1 and HIV-2 in female sex workers in Abidjan, Cote d'Ivoire. *AIDS, 9,* 955–958.

Gleeson, M. C. (1996). High-risk sexual behavior in college students: An examination of antecedents from childhood maltreatment. Unpublished doctoral dissertation, University of Connecticut, Storrs.

Gleeson, M. K., & Becker-Lausen, E. (1996, August). *Vulnerability to risky sexual behavior: Child maltreatment, externality, and dissociation.* Poster presentation, 104th Annual Convention of the American Psychological Association, Toronto.

Gordon, C. P. (1996). Adolescent decision making: A broadly based theory and its application to the prevention of early pregnancy. *Adolescence, 31,* 561–584.

Gourevitch, M. N., Hartel, D., Schoenbaum, E. E., Selwyn, P. A., Davenny, K., Friedland, G. H., & Klein, R. S. (1996). A prospective study of syphilis and HIV infection among injection drug users receiving methadone in the Bronx, NY. *American Journal of Public Health, 86,* 1112–1115.

Graham, C. A. (1994). AIDS and the adolescent. *International Journal of STD and AIDS, 5,* 305–309.

Graham, J. R. (1993). *MMPI-2: Assessing personality and psychopathology* (2nd ed.). New York: Oxford.

Grimley, D. M., Riley, G. E., Bellis, J. M., & Prochaska, J. O. (1993). Assessing the Stages of Change and decision-making for contraceptive use for the prevention of pregnancy, sexually transmitted diseases, and Acquired Immunodeficiency Syndrome. *Health Education Quarterly, 20,* 455–470.

Gunn, R. A., Montes, J. M., Toomey, K. E., Rolfs, R. T., Greenspan, J. R., Spitters, C. E., & Waterman, S. H. (1995). Syphilis in San Diego County 1983–1992: Crack cocaine, prostitution, and the limitations of partner notification. *Sexually Transmitted Diseases, 22,* 60–66.

Hamers, F. F., Peterman, T. A., Zaidi, A. A., Ransom, R. L., Wroten, J. E., & Witte, J. J. (1995). Syphilis and gonorrhea in Miami: Similar clustering, different trends. *American Journal of Public Health, 85,* 1104–1108.

Hankin, J. R. (1996). Alcohol warning labels: Influence on drinking. In Abel, E. L. (Ed.), *Fetal alcohol syndrome: From mechanism to prevention* (pp. 27–50). Boca Raton, FL: CRC Press.

Hart, G. J., Dawsen, J., Fitzpatrick, R. M., Boulton, M., McLean, J., Brookes, M., & Parry, J. V. (1993). Risk behaviour, anti-HIV and anti-hepatitis B core prevalence in clinic and non-clinic samples of gay men in England, 1991–1992. *AIDS, 7,* 863–869.

Hawkins, W. E., Spigner, C., & Murphy, M. (1990). Perceived use of health education services in a school-based clinic. *Perceptual and Motor Skills, 70,* 1075–1078.

Heckman, T. G., Kelly, J. A., Sikkema, K. J., Roffman, R. R., Solomon, L. J., Winett, R. A., Stevenson, L. Y., Perry, M. J., Norman, A. D., & Desiderato, L. J. (1995). Differences in HIV risk characteristics between bisexual and exclusively gay men. *AIDS Education and Prevention, 7,* 504–512.

Hein, K. (1992). Adolescents at risk for HIV acquisition. In R. DiClemente (Ed.), *Adolescents: A generation in jeopardy* (pp. 3–16). Newbury Park, CA: Sage.

Herek, G. M. (1993). Documenting prejudice against lesbians and gay men on campus: The Yale Sexual Orientation Survey. *Journal of Homosexuality, 25* (4), 15–30.

Herman, J. L., & van der Kolk, B. A. (1987). Traumatic antecedents of Borderline Personality Disorder. In B. A. van der Kolk (Ed.), *Psychological trauma* (pp. 111–126). Washington, DC: American Psychiatric Press.

Herrmann, B., & Egger, M. (1995). Genital chlamydia trachomatis infections in Uppsala County, Sweden, 1985–1993: Declining rates for how much longer? *Sexually Transmitted Diseases, 22,* 253–260.

Hiatt, S. W., Sampson, D., & Baird, D. (1997). Paraprofessional home visitation: Conceptual and pragmatic considerations. *Journal of Community Psychology, 25,* 77–93.

Hickson, F. C.I., Reid, D. S., Davies, P. M., Weatherburn, P., Beardsell, S., & Keogh, P. G. (1996). No aggregate change in homosexual HIV risk behaviour among gay men attending the Gay Pride festivals, United Kingdom, 1993–1995. *AIDS, 10,* 771–774.

Hillard, D., Shank, J. C., & Redman, R. W. (1982). Unplanned pregnancies in a midwestern community. *Journal of Family Practice, 15,* 259–263.

Hillard, P. J. (1992). Oral contraception noncompliance: The extent of the problem. *Advances in Contraception,* 8, 13–20.

Hoisen, J. H. (1993). Healing from cultural victimization: Recovery from shame due to heterosexism. *Journal of Gay and Lesbian Psychotherapy, 2* (1), 49–63.

Holmes, G. R., Offen, L., & Waller, G. (1997). See no evil, hear no evil, speak no evil: Why do relatively few male victims of childhood sexual abuse receive help for abuse-related issues in adulthood? *Clinical Psychology Review, 17* (1), 69–88.

Holmes, K. K., Karon, J. M., Kreiss, J. (1990). The increasing frequency of heterosexually acquired AIDS in the United States, 1983–88. *American Journal of Public Health, 80,* 858–862.

Hooper, C. A. (1989). Alternatives to collusion: The response of mothers to child sexual abuse in the family. *Educational and Child Psychology, 6* (1), 22–30.

Hoppe, M. J., Wells, E. A., Wilsdon, A., Gillmore, M. R., & Morrison, D. M. (1994). Children's knowledge and beliefs about AIDS: Qualitative data from focus group interviews. *Health Education Quarterly, 21* (1), 117–126.

Hunter, J. (1990). Violence against lesbian and gay male youths. *Journal of Interpersonal Violence, 5,* 295–300.

Hunter, J. A. (1991). A comparison of the psychosocial maladjustment of adult males and females sexually molested as children. *Journal of Interpersonal Violence, 6,* 205–217.

Icard, L. D., Schilling, R. F., el Bassel, N., & Young, D. (1992). Preventing AIDS among black gay men and black gay and heterosexual male intravenous drug users. *Social Work, 37,* 440–445.

Inciardi, J. A. (1995). Crack, crack house sex, and HIV risk. *Archives of Sexual Behavior, 24* (3), 249–269.

Indian Council of Medical Research Task Force on IUD and Hormonal Contraceptives. (1994). Improved utilization of spacing methods—intrauterine devices (IUDs) and low-dose combined oral contraceptives (OCs)—through re-orientation training for improving quality of services. *Contraception, 50* (3), 215–228.

Indian Health Service (1990). *AIDS prevention activity.* Phoenix, AZ: Clinical Support Center, 4412 N. 16th Street.

James, J., & Meyerding, J. (1977). Early sexual experiences and prostitution. *American Journal of Psychiatry, 134,* 1381–1385.

Jemmott, J. B., Jemmott, L. S., & Fong, G. T. (1992). Reduction in HIV risk—Associated sexual behaviors among black male adolescents: Effects of an AIDS prevention intervention. *American Journal of Public Health, 82,* 372–377.

Jessor, S., & Jessor, R. (1975). Transition from virginity to nonvirginity among youth: A social-psychological study over time. *Developmental Psychology, 11,* 473–484.

John, G. C., & Kreiss, J. (1996). Mother-to-child transmission of human immunodeficiency virus type 1. *Epidemiologic Reviews, 18* (2), 149–157.

Johnstone, H., Tornabene, M., & Marcinak, J. (1993). Incidence of sexually transmitted diseases and Pap smear results in female homeless clients from the Chicago Health Outreach Project. *Health Care for Women International, 14,* 293–299.

Jones, C. L. (1996). Herpes simplex virus infection in the neonate: Clinical presentation and management. *Neonatal Network: Journal of Neonatal Nursing, 15* (8), 11–15, 22–24.

Jones, D. C., Rickel, A. U., & Smith, R. L. (1980). Maternal child rearing practices and social problem solving strategies among preschoolers. *Developmental Psychology, 16,* 241–242.

Jonna, S., Collins, M., Abedin, M., Young, M., Milteer, R., & Beeram, M. (1995). Postneonatal screening for congenital syphilis. *Journal of Family Practice, 41,* 286–288.

Kalichman, S. C. (1995). *Understanding AIDS: A guide for mental health professionals.* Washington, DC: American Psychological Association.

Kalichman, S. C., & Rompa, D. (1995). Sexually coerced and noncoerced gay and bisexual men: Factors relevant to risk for Human Immunodeficiency Virus (HIV) infection. *Journal of Sex Research, 32,* 45–50.

Kalichman, S. C., Kelly, J. A., & St. Lawrence, J. S. (1990). Factors influencing reduction of sexual risk behaviors for human immunodeficiency virus infection: A review. *Annals of Sex Research, 3,* 129–148.

Kalichman, S. C., Hunter, T., & Kelly, J. (1992). Perceptions of AIDS risk susceptibility among minority and nonminority women at risk for HIV infection. *Journal of Consulting and Clinical Psychology, 60,* 725–732.

Kalichman, S. C., Kelly, J. A., Hunter, T. L., Murphy, D. A., & Tyler, R. (1993). Culturally tailored HIV-AIDS risk-reduction messages targeted to African-American urban women: Impact on risk sensitization and risk reduction. *Journal of Consulting and Clinical Psychology, 61,* 291–295.

Kalichman, S. C., Adair, V., Somlai, A. M., & Weir, S. S. (1995). The perceived social context of AIDS: Study of inner-city sexually transmitted disease clinic patients. *AIDS Education and Prevention, 7,* 298–307.

Kantor, D., Peretz, A., & Zander, R. (1984). The cycle of poverty: Where to begin? *Family Therapy Collections, 9,* 59–73.

Kaufman, J., & Zigler, E. (1987). Do abused children become abusive parents? *American Journal of Orthopsychiatry, 57,* 186–192.

Kegeles, S. M., Adler, N. E., & Irwin, C. E. (1988). Sexually active adolescents and condoms: Changes over one year in knowledge, attitudes, and use. *American Journal of Public Health, 78,* 460–461.

Kelly, J. A., & Murphy, D. A. (1991). Some lessons learned about risk reduction after ten years of the HIV/AIDS epidemic. *AIDS Care, 3,* 251–257.

Kelly, J. A., St. Lawrence, J. S., & Brasfield, T. L. (1991). Predictors of vulnerability to AIDS risk behavior relapse. *Journal of Consulting and Clinical Psychology, 59,* 163–166.

Kelly, J. A., St. Lawrence, J. S., Diaz, Y. E., Stevenson, L. Y., Hauth, A. C., Brasfield, T. L., Kalichman, S. C., Smith, J. E., & Andrew, M. E. (1991). HIV risk behavior reduction following intervention with key opinion leaders of population: An experimental analysis. *American Journal of Public Health, 81,* 168–171.

Kelly, J. A., St. Lawrence, J. S., Stevenson, L. Y., Hauth, A. C., Kalichman, S. C., Diaz, Y. E., Brasfield, T. L., Koob, J. J., & Morgan, M. G. (1992). Community AIDS/HIV risk reduction: The effects of endorsements by popular people in three cities. *American Journal of Public Health, 82,* 1483–1489.

Kelly, J. A., Sikkema, K. J., Winett, R. A., Solomon, L. J., Roffman, R. A., Heckman, T. G., Stevenson, L. Y., Perry, M. J., Norman, A. D., & Desiderato, L. J. (1995). Factors predicting continued high-risk behavior among gay men in small cities: Psychological, behavioral, and demographic characteristics related to unsafe sex. *Journal of Consulting and Clinical Psychology, 63,* 101–107.

Kemeny, M. E., Weiner, H., Duran, R., Taylor, S. E., Visscher, B., & Fahey, J. L. (1995). Immune system changes after the death of a partner in HIV-positive gay men. *Psychosomatic Medicine, 57,* 547–554.

Kenney, J. W. (1996). Risk factors associated with genital HPV infection. *Cancer Nursing, 19,* 353–359.

Kilpatrick, D. G., Veronen, L. J., Saunders, B. E., Best, C. L., Amick-McMullen, A., & Paduhovich, J. (1987, March). *The psychological impact of crime: A study of randomly surveyed crime victims* (Final report, grant #84-IJ-CX-0039). Washington, DC: National Institute of Justice.

Kilpatrick, D. G., Edmunds, C. N., & Seymour, A. K. (1992). *Rape in America: A report to the nation.* Arlington, VA: National Victim Center.

Kirby, D., Barth, R. P., Leland, N., & Fetro, J. V. (1991). Reducing the risk: Impact of a new curriculum on sexual risk-taking. *Family Planning Perspectives, 23,* 253–263.

Kitamura, T., Shima, S., Sugawara, M., & Toda, M. A. (1993). Psychological and social correlates of the onset of affective disorders among pregnant women. *Psychological Medicine, 23,* 967–975.

Kitzman, H. J., Cole, R., Yoos, H. L., & Olds, D. (1997). Challenges experienced by home visitors: A qualitative study of program implementation. *Journal of Community Psychology, 25,* 95–109.

Kluft, R. P. (1990a). Dissociation and subsequent vulnerability: A preliminary study. *Dissociation, 3* (3), 167–173.

Kluft, R. P. (1990b). Editorial: The darker side of dissociation. *Dissociation, 3* (3), 125.

Koniak-Griffin, D., & Brecht, M. L. (1995). Linkages between sexual risk taking, substance use, and AIDS knowledge among pregnant adolescents and young mothers. *Nursing Research, 44,* 340–346.

Koss, M. P. (1993). Detecting the scope of rape: A review of prevalence research methods. *Journal of Interpersonal Violence, 8* (2), 198–222.

Koss, M. P., Dinero, T. E., Seibel, C. A., & Cox, S. L. (1988). Stranger and acquaintance rape: Are there differences in the victims experience? *Psychology of Women Quarterly, 12,* 1–24.

Krieger, J. N. (1995). Trichomoniasis in men: Old issues and new data. *Sexually Transmitted Diseases, 22* (2), 83–96.

Krieger, J. N., Verdon, M., Siegel, N., Critchlow, C., & Holmes, K. K. (1992). Risk assessment and laboratory diagnosis of trichomoniasis in men. *Journal of Infectious Diseases, 166,* 1362–1366.

Kubicka, L., Matejcek, Z., David, H. P., Dytrych, Z., Miller, W. B., & Roth, Z. (1995). Children from unwanted pregnancies in Prague, Czech Republic revisited at age thirty. *Acta Psychiatrica Scandinavica, 91,* 361–369.

Leigh, B. C. (1990). The relationship of substance use during sex to high-risk sexual behavior. *Journal of Sex Research, 27* (2), 199–213.

Lemp, G. F., Jones, M., Kellogg, T. A., Nieri, G. N., Anderson, L., Withum, D., & Katz, M. (1995). HIV seroprevalence and risk behaviors among lesbians and bisexual women in San Francisco and Berkeley, California. *American Journal of Public Health, 85,* 1549–1552.

Lennon, M. C., Martin, J. L., & Dean, L. (1990). The influence of social support on AIDS-related grief reaction among gay men. *Social Science and Medicine, 31,* 477–484.

Lewin, T. (1997, October 1). Sexual abuse tied to 1 in 4 girls in teens: Later harm is also traced in 2 studies. *New York Times,* A24.

Lisak, D. (1994). The psychological impact of sexual abuse: Content analysis of interviews with male survivors. *Journal of Traumatic Stress, 7,* 525–548.

Longshore, D., & Anglin, M. D. (1995). Number of sex partners and crack cocaine use: Is crack an independent marker for HIV risk behavior? *The Journal of Drug Issues, 25* (1), 1–10.

Maier, S. E., Chen, W. J. A., & West, J. R. (1996). The effects of timing and duration of alcohol exposure on the development of the fetal brain. In Abel, E. L. (Ed.) *Fetal alcohol syndrome: From mechanism to prevention* (pp. 27–50). Boca Raton, FL: CRC Press.

Mann, J., Tarantola, D. J.M., & Neter, T. W. (Eds.). (1992). *AIDS in the world.* Cambridge, MA: Harvard University Press.

Manteuffel, M. D. (1996). Neurotransmitter function: Changes associated with in utero alcohol exposure. In E. L. Abel (Ed.) *Fetal alcohol syndrome: From mechanism to prevention* (pp. 171–189). Boca Raton, FL: CRC Press.

Marin, B. V., & Gomez, C. A. (1997). Latino culture and sex: Implications for HIV prevention. In J. G. Garcia & M. C. Zea (Eds.), *Psychological interventions and research with Latino populations* (pp. 73–93). Boston: Allyn and Bacon.

Marin, B. V., Gomez, C. A., & Hearst, N. (1993). Multiple heterosexual partners and condom use among Hispanics and non-Hispanic whites. *Family Planning Perspectives, 25,* 170–174.

Marin, B. V., Gomez, C. A., & Tschann, J. (1993). Condom use with casual partners with secondary female sexual partners. *Public Health Reports, 108,* 742–750.

Marin, B. V., Tschann, J., Gomez, C., & Kegeles, S. (1993). Acculturation and gender differences in sexual attitudes and behaviors: A comparison of Hispanic and non-Hispanic white single adults. *American Journal of Public Health, 83,* 1759–1761.

Marsiglio, W. (1989). Adolescent males' pregnancy resolution preferences and family formation intentions: Does family background make a difference for blacks and whites? *Journal of Adolescent Research, 4* (2), 214–237.

Martin, D. J. (1993). Coping with AIDS and AIDS-risk reduction efforts among gay men. *AIDS Education and Prevention, 5,* 104–120.

Martin, H. L., Jr., Stevens, C. E., Richardson, B. A., Rugamba, D., Nyange, P. M., Mandaliya, K., Ndinya-Achola, J., & Kreiss, J. K. (1997). Safety of nonoxynol-9 vaginal gel in Kenyan prostitutes. A randomized clinical trial. *Sexually Transmitted Diseases, 24,* 279–283.

Martin, J. L., & Dean, L. (1993). Effects of AIDS-related bereavement and HIV-related illness on psychological distress among gay men: A 7-year longitudinal study, 1985–1991. *Journal of Consulting and Clinical Psychology, 61,* 94–103.

McFarlin, B. L., & Bottoms, S. F. (1995). Maternal syphilis in Michigan: The challenge to prevent congenital syphilis. *Midwifery, 11* (2), 55–60.

McKusick, L., Hoff, C. C., Stall, R., & Coates, T. J. (1991). Tailoring AIDS prevention: Differences in behavioral strategies among heterosexual and gay bar patrons in San Francisco. *AIDS Education and Prevention, 3,* 1–9.

McLanahan, S., & Sandefur, G. (1994). *Growing up with a single parent.* Cambridge, MA: Harvard University Press.

Meyer, I. H., & Dean, L. (1995). Patterns of sexual behavior and risk taking among young New York City gay men. *AIDS Education and Prevention, 7,* Supplement, 13–23.

Millan, F., & Caban, M. (1996). Issues in psychotherapy with HIV-infected Latinos in New York City. *Journal of Social Distress and the Homeless, 5* (1), 83–98.

Miller, B., & Marshall, J. C. (1987). Coercive sex on the university campus. *Journal of College Student Personnel, 28* (1), 38–47.

Miller, J., Moeller, D., Kaufman, A., Divasto, P., Fitzsimmons, P., Pather, D, & Christy, J. (1978). Recidivism among sexual assault victims. *American Journal of Psychiatry, 135,* 1103–1104.

Miller, W. R., & Rollnick, S. (1991). *Motivational interviewing: Preparing people to change addictive behavior.* New York: The Guilford Press.

Moskowitz, J. T., Folkman, S., Collette, L., & Vittinghoff, E. (1996). Coping and mood during AIDS-related caregiving and bereavement. *Annals of Behavioral Medicine, 18* (1), 49–57.

Mulry, G., Kalichman, S. C., & Kelly, J. A. (1994). Substance use and unsafe sex among gay men: Global versus situational use of substances. *Journal of Sex Education and Therapy, 20,* 175–184.

Murphy, P. A., & Jones, E. (1994). Use of oral metronidazole in pregnancy: Risks, benefits, and practice guidelines. *Journal of Nurse Midwifery, 39,* 214–220.

Murry, V. M. (1995). An ecological analysis of pregnancy resolution decisions among African American and Hispanic adolescent females. *Youth and Society, 26,* 325–350.

Najman, J. M., Morrison, J., Williams, G., Andersen, M., & Keeping, J. D. (1991). The mental health of women 6 months after they give birth to an unwanted baby: A longitudinal study. *Social Science and Medicine, 32,* 241–247.

Nakou, S., Adam, H., Stathacopoulou, N., & Agathonos, H. (1982). Health status of abused and neglected children and their siblings. *Child Abuse and Neglect, 6,* 279–284.

Nash, M. R., Hulsey, T. L., Sexton, M. C., Harralson, T. L., & Lambert, W. (1993). Long-term sequelae of childhood sexual abuse: Perceived family environment, psychopathology, and dissociation. *Journal of Consulting and Clinical Psychology, 61,* 276–283.

Neisen, J. H. (1993). Parental substance abuse and divorce as predictors of injection drug use and high risk sexual behaviors known to transmit HIV. *Journal of Psychology and Human Sexuality, 6* (2), 29–49.

Neisen, J. H., & Sandall, H. (1990). Alcohol and other drug abuse in a gay/lesbian population: Related to victimization? *Journal of Psychology and Human Sexuality, 3* (1), 151–168.

Ney, P. G., Fung, T., Wickett, A. R., & Beaman-Dodd, C. (1994). The effects of pregnancy loss on women's health. *Social Science and Medicine, 38,* 1193–1200.

Nord, D. (1996). Issues and implications in the counseling of survivors of multiple AIDS-related loss. *Death Studies, 20,* 389–413.

Offir, J. T., Fisher, J. D., Williams, S. S., & Fisher, W. A. (1993). Reasons for inconsistent AIDS-preventive behaviors among gay men. *Journal of Sex Research, 30,* 62–69.

Oh, M. K., Cloud, G. A., Fleenor, M., Sturdevant, M. S., Nesmith, J. D., & Feinstein, R. A. (1996). Risk for gonococcal and chlamydial cervicitis in adolescent females: Incidence and recurrence in a prospective cohort study. *Journal of Adolescent Health, 18,* 270–275.

Oliver, J. E. (1993). Intergenerational transmission of child abuse: Rates, research, and clinical implications. *American Journal of Psychiatry, 150,* 1315–1324.

Onorato, I. M., O'Brien, T. R., Schable, C. A., Spruill, C., & Holmberg, S. D. (1993). Sentinel surveillance for HIV-2 infection in high-risk U. S. populations. *American Journal of Public Health, 83,* 515–519.

Osmond, M. W., Wambach, K. G., Harrison, D. F., Byers, J., Levine, P., Imershein, A., & Quadagno, D. M. (1993). The multiple jeopardy of race, class, and gender for AIDS risk among women. *Gender and Society, 7* (1), 99–120.

Paul, J. P., Stall, R., & Bloomfield, K. A. (1991). Gay and alcoholic: Epidemiologic and clinical issues. *Alcohol Health and Research World, 15,* 151–160.

Paul, J. P., Stall, R., & Davis, F. (1993). Sexual risk for HIV transmission among gay/bisexual men in substance-abuse treatment. *AIDS Education and Prevention, 5,* 11–24.

Peluso, E., & Putnam, N. (1996). Case study: Sexual abuse of boys by females. *Journal of the American Academy of Child and Adolescent Psychiatry, 35* (1), 51–54.

Perkins, D. O., Leserman, J., Murphy, C., & Evans, D. L. (1993). Psychosocial predictors of high-risk sexual behavior among HIV-negative homosexual men. *AIDS Education and Prevention, 5* (2), 141–152.

Perry, M. J., Solomon, L. J., Winett, R. A., Kelly, J. A., Roffman, R. A., Desiderato, L. L., Kalichman, S. C., Sikkema, K. J., Norman, A. D., Short, B., & Stevenson, L. Y. (1994). High risk sexual behavior and alcohol consumption among bar-going gay men. *AIDS, 8,* 1321–1324.

Peterson, J. L., Coates, T. J., Catania, J. A., Middleton, L., Hilliard, B., & Hearst, N. (1992). High-risk sexual behavior and condom use among gay and bisexual African-American men. *American Journal of Public Health, 82,* 1490–1494.

Phillips, A., & Johnson, A. (1992). Female-to-male transmission of HIV. *JAMA, 268,* 1855–1856.

Prinos, M. J. (1996). Intergenerational patterns of psychological maltreatment, child rearing practices, and trauma-related symptomatology in a clinical population. Unpublished doctoral dissertation, University of Connecticut, Storrs.

Prinos, M. J., Becker-Lausen, E., & Rickel, A. U. (1997, August). *Measurement of parental practices: Nurturance, restrictiveness, inconsistency, and child maltreatment.* Poster presentation, 105th Annual Convention of the American Psychological Association, Chicago.

Prochaska, J. O. (1994). Strong and weak principles for progressing from precontemplation to action on the basis of twelve problem behaviors. *Health Psychology, 13,* 47–51.

Prochaska, J. O., & DiClemente, C. C. (1982). Transtheoretical therapy: Toward a more integrative model of change. *Psychotherapy: Theory, Research and Practice, 20,* 161–173.

Prochaska, J. O., & DiClemente, C. C. (1984). *The transtheoretical approach: Crossing traditional boundaries of change.* Homewood, IL: Dorsey Press.

Prochaska, J. O., Diclemente, C. C., & Norcross, J. C. (1992). In search of how people change: Applications to addictive behaviors. *American Psychologist, 47,* 1102–1114.

Prochaska, J. O., Velicer, W. F., Rossi, J. S., Goldstein, M. G., Marcus, B. H., Rakowski, W., Fiore, C., Harlow, L. L., Redding, C. A., Rosenbloom, D., & Rossi, S. R. (1994). Stages of change and decisional balance for 12 problem behaviors. *Health Psychology, 13,* 39–46.

Rabin, J. M., Seltzer, V., & Pollack, S. (1991). The long-term benefits of a comprehensive teenage pregnancy program. *Clinical Pediatrics, 30,* 305–309.

Ramirez, J., Suarez, E., de la Rosa, G., Castro, M. A., & Zimmerman, M. A. (1994). AIDS knowledge and sexual behavior among Mexican gay and bisexual men. *AIDS Education and Prevention, 6,* 163–174.

Rankin, E., & Becker-Lausen, E. (1997, June). *Further validation of the Child Abuse and Trauma (CAT) scale: MMPI data.* Poster presentation, Family Research Consortium Summer Institute, San Antonio, TX.

Remien, R. H., Goetz, R., Rabkin, J. G., Williams, J. B.W., Bradbury, M., Ehrhardt, A. A., & Gorman, J. M. (1995). Remission of substance use disorders: Gay men in the first decade of AIDS. *Journal of Studies on Alcohol, 56,* 226–232.

Resick, P. A. (1993). The psychological impact of rape. *Journal of Interpersonal Violence, 8,* 223–255.

Resick, P. A., & Schnicke, M. K. (1992). Cognitive processing therapy for sexual assault victims. *Journal of Consulting and Clinical Psychology, 60,* 748–756.

Resick, P. A., & Schnicke, M. K. (1993). *Cognitive processing therapy for rape victims: A treatment manual.* Newbury Park, CA: Sage.

Rice, R. J., Roberts, P. L., Handsfield, H. H., & Holmes, K. K. (1991). Sociodemographic distribution of gonorrhea incidence: Implications for prevention and behavioral research. *American Journal of Public Health, 81,* 1252–1258.

Rickel, A. U. (1989). *Teen pregnancy and parenting.* New York: Hemisphere Publishing Corporation.

Rickel, A. U., & Becker, E. (1997). *Keeping children from harm's way.* Washington, DC: American Psychological Association.

Rickel, A. U., & Becker-Lausen, E. (1994). Treating the adolescent drug misuser. In T. P. Gullotta, G. R. Adams, & R. Montemayor (Eds.), *Substance misuse in adolescence* (pp. 175–200. Thousand Oaks, CA: Sage.

Rickel, A. U., & Becker-Lausen, E. (1995). Intergenerational influences on child outcomes: Implications for prevention and intervention. In B. A. Ryan, G. R. Adams, T. P. Gullotta, R. P. Weissberg, & R. L. Hampton (Eds.), *The family-school connection: Theory, research, and practice* (pp. 315–340). Thousand Oaks, CA: Sage.

Rickel, A. U., & Biasatti, L. L. (1982). Modification of the Block Child Rearing Practices Report. *Journal of Clinical Psychology, 38,* 129–134.

Rickel, A. U., Dudley, G., & Berman, S. (1980). An evaluation of parent training. *Evaluation Review, 4,* 389–403.

Rodgers, J. L., & Rowe, D. C. (1993). Social contagion and adolescent sexual behavior: A developmental EMOSA model. *Psychological Review, 100,* 479–510.

Rogers, M. F., & Kilbourne, B. W. (1992). Epidemiology of pediatric HIV infection. In G. P. Wormser (Ed.), *AIDS and other manifestations of HIV infection* (2nd. ed., pp. 17–24). New York: Raven Press.

Roper, W. L., Peterson, H. B., & Curran, J. W. (1993). Commentary: Condoms and HIV/STD prevention—Clarifying the message. *American Journal of Public Health, 83,* 501–503.

Roth, S., Wayland, K., & Woolsey, M. (1990). Victimization history and victim-assailant relationship as factors in recovery from sexual assault. *Journal of Traumatic Stress, 3* (1), 169–180.

Rothbaum, B. O., Foa, E. B., Murdock, T., Riggs, D. S., & Walsh, W. (1992). A prospective examination of post-traumatic stress disorder in rape victims. *Journal of Traumatic Stress, 5,* 455–475.

Rotheram-Borus, M. J., & Koopman, C. (1991). HIV and adolescents. *Journal of Primary Prevention, 12* (1), 65–82.

Rotter, J. B. (1954/1980). *Social learning theory and clinical psychology.* New York: Johnson Reprint Company.

Rotter, J. B. (1966). Generalized expectancies for internal versus external control of reinforcement. *Psychological Monographs, 80* (1, Whole No. 609).

Rowe, P. M. (1997). Nonoxynol-9 fails to protect against HIV-1. *Lancet, 349,* 1074.

Ruch-Ross, H. S., Jones, E. D., & Musick, J. S. (1992). Comparing outcomes in a statewide program for adolescent mothers with outcomes in a national sample. *Family Planning Perspectives, 24,* 66–71.

Runtz, M., & Briere, J. (1986). Adolescent "acting out" and childhood history of sexual abuse. *Journal of Interpersonal Violence, 1,* 326–334.

Russell, D. E. H. (1986). *The secret trauma: Incest in the lives of girls and women.* New York: Basic Books.

Russo, N. F., & Zierk, K. L. (1992). Abortion, childbearing, and women's well-being. *Professional Psychology: Research and Practice, 23,* 269–280.

Russo, N. F., Horn, J. D., & Schwartz, R. (1992). U. S. abortion in context: Selected characteristics and motivations of women seeking abortions. *Journal of Social Issues, 48* (3), 183–202.

Sabogal, F., Perez-Stable, E. J., Otero-Sabogal, R., & Hiatt, R. A. (1995). Gender, ethnic, and acculturation differences in sexual behaviors: Hispanic and non-Hispanic White adults. *Hispanic Journal of the Behavioral Sciences, 17* (2), 139–159.

Sandberg, G., Jackson, T. L., & Petretic-Jackson, P. (1987). College students' attitudes regarding sexual coercion and aggression: Developing educational and preventive strategies. *Journal of College Student Personnel, 28,* 302–311.

Sanders, B., & Becker-Lausen, E. (1995). The measurement of psychological maltreatment: Early data on the Child Abuse and Trauma scale. *Child Abuse and Neglect, 19,* 315–323.

Savin-Williams, R. C. (1994). Verbal and physical abuse as stressors in the lives of lesbian, gay male, and bisexual youths: Associations with school problems, running away, substance abuse, prostitution, and suicide. *Journal of Consulting and Clinical Psychology, 62,* 261–269.

Segest, E. (1994). Some aspects regarding teenage pregnancy in Denmark. *Medicine and the Law, 13,* 381–396.

Seibt, A. C., Ross, M. W., Freeman, A., Krepcho, M., Hedrich, A., McAlister, A., & Fernandez-Esquer, M. E. (1995). Relationship between safe sex and acculturation into the gay subculture. *AIDS Care, 7* (Supplement 1), S85-S88.

Seidman, S. N., Mosher, W. D., & Aral, S. O. (1992). Women with multiple sex partners: United States, 1988. *American Journal of Public Health, 82,* 1388–1394.

Seitz, V., & Apfel, N. H. (1993). Adolescent mothers and repeated childbearing: Effects of a school-based intervention program. *American Journal of Orthopsychiatry, 63,* 572–581.

Selik, R. M., Castro, K. G., & Pappaioanou, M. (1988). Racial/ethnic differences in risk of AIDS. *American Journal of Public Health, 78,* 1539–1545.

Sellers, D. E., McGraw, S. A., McKinlay, J. B. (1994). Does the promotion and distribution of condoms increase teen sexual activity? Evidence from an HIV prevention program for Latino youth. *American Journal of Public Health, 84* (12), 1952–1959.

Shapiro, B. L., & Schwarz, J. C. (1997). Date rape: Its relationship to trauma symptoms and sexual self-esteem. *Journal of Interpersonal Violence, 12* (3), 407–419.

Shealy, C. N. (1995). From *Boys Town* to *Oliver Twist:* Separating fact from fiction in welfare reform and out-of-home placement of children and youth. *American Psychologist, 50,* 565–580.

Shernoff, M., & Finnegan, D. (1991). Family treatment with chemically dependent gay men and lesbians. *Journal of Chemical Dependency Treatment, 4* (1), 121–135.

Shifrin, F., & Solis, M. (1992). Chemical dependency in gay and lesbian youth. *Journal of Chemical Dependency Treatment, 5* (1), 67–76.

Shoop, D. M., & Davidson, P. M. (1994). AIDS and adolescents: The relation of parent and partner communication to adolescent condom use. *Journal of Adolescence, 17* (2), 137–148.

Sidel, R. (1996). *Keeping women and children last.* New York: Penguin Books.

Siegel, K., & Krauss, B. J. (1991). Living with HIV infection: Adaptive tasks of seropositive gay men. *Journal of Health and Social Behavior, 32* (1), 17–32.

Sikkema, K. J., Winett, R. A., & Lombard, D. N. (1995). Development and evaluation of an HIV-risk reduction program for female college students. *AIDS Education and Prevention, 7* (2), 145–159.

Sitzman, B. T., Burch, E. A., Jr., Bartlett, L. S., & Urrutia, G. (1995). Rates of sexually transmitted diseases among patients in a psychiatric emergency service. *Psychiatric Services, 46,* 136–140.

Skinner, W. F. (1994). The prevalence and demographic predictors of illicit and licit drug use among lesbians and gay men. *American Journal of Public Health, 84,* 1307–1310.

Smith, C., & Thornberry, T. (1995). The relationship between childhood maltreatment and adolescent involvement in delinquency. *Criminology, 33,* 451–481.

Smith, C., Lizotte, A. J., Thornberry, T. P., & Krohn, M. D. (1995). Resilient youth: Identifying factors that prevent high-risk youth from engaging in delinquency and drug use. *Current Perspectives on Aging and the Life Cycle, 4,* 217–247.

Speckhard, A. C., & Rue, V. M. (1992). Postabortion syndrome: An emerging public health concern. *Journal of Social Issues, 48* (3), 95–119.

Steiner, M., Foldesy, R., Cole, D., & Carter, E. (1992). Study to determine the correlation between condom breakage in human use and laboratory test results. *Contraception, 46,* 279–288.

Steiner, M., Piedrahita, C., Glover, L., Joanis, C., Spruyt, A., & Foldesy, R. (1994). The impact of lubricants on latex condoms during vaginal intercourse. *International Journal of STD and AIDS, 5* (1), 29–36.

Stevenson, H. C., & Davis, G. (1994). Impact of culturally sensitive AIDS video education on the AIDS risk knowledge of African-American adolescents. *AIDS Education and Prevention, 6* (1), 40–52.

Stevenson, H. C., & White, J. (1990). *Barriers to AIDS education and prevention in minority communities: Making the best of a grave situation.* Unpublished manuscript. Philadelphia: Philadelphia Refugee Service Center.

Stewart, B. D., Hughes, C., Frank, E., Anderson, B. Kendall, K., & West, D. (1987). Profiles of immediate and delayed treatment seekers. *Journal of Nervous and Mental Disease, 175,* 90–94.

St. Lawrence, J. S. (1993). African-American adolescents' knowledge, health-related attitudes, sexual behavior, and contraceptive decisions: Implications for the prevention of adolescent HIV infection. *Journal of Consulting and Clinical Psychology, 61,* 104–112.

Stratton, P., & Alexander, N. J. (1993). Prevention of sexually transmitted infections. Physical and chemical barrier methods. *Infectious Disease Clinics of North America, 7,* 841–859.

Sullivan, M. L. (1993). Culture and class as determinants of out-of-wedlock childbearing and poverty during late adolescence. *Journal of Research on Adolescence, 3,* 295–316.

Susser, I., & Gonzalez, M. A. (1992). Sex, drugs and videotape: The prevention of AIDS in a New York City shelter for homeless men. *Medical Anthropology, 14,* 307–322.

Swanson, J. M., Dibble, S. L., & Chenitz, W. C. (1995). Clinical features and psychosocial factors in young adults with genital herpes. *Image: Journal of Nursing Scholarship, 27* (1), 16–22.

Sweat, M. D., & Levin, M. (1995). HIV/AIDS knowledge among the U. S. population. *AIDS Education and Prevention, 7,* 355–375.

Thomas, E. A., & Rickel, A. U. (1995). Teen pregnancy and maladjustment: A study of base rates. *Journal of Community Psychology, 23,* 200–215.

Thomas, J. C., Schoenbach, V. J., Weiner, D. H., Parker, E. A., & Earp, J. A. (1996). Rural gonorrhea in the southeastern United States: A neglected epidemic? *American Journal of Epidemiology, 143,* 269–277.

Thompson, B. L., Matuszak, D., Dwyer, D. M., Nakashima, A., Pearce, H., & Israel, E. (1995). Congenital syphilis in Maryland, 1989–1991: The effect of changing the case definition and opportunities for prevention. *Sexually Transmitted Diseases, 22,* 364–369.

U. S. Advisory Board on Child Abuse and Neglect. (1995). *A nation's shame: Fatal child abuse and neglect in the United States. A report of the U. S. Advisory Board on Child Abuse and Neglect.* Washington, DC: U. S. Department of Health and Human Services.

U. S. Department of Health and Human Services. (1994). *Evaluation and management of early HIV infection.* (AHCPR Publication No. 94–0572). Rockville, MD: Author.

U. S. Public Health Service. (1993, February/March). *Prevention report.* Washington, DC: U. S. Department of Health and Human Services.

van der Kolk, B. A. (1989). The compulsion to repeat the trauma: Re-enactment, revictimization, and masochism. *Psychiatric Clinics of North America, 12,* 389–411.

van der Kolk, B. A. (1996). The complexity of adaptation to trauma: Self-regulation, stimulus discrimination, and characterological development. In B. A. van der Kolk, A. C. McFarlane, & L. Weisaeth (Eds.), *Traumatic stress: The effects of overwhelming experience on mind, body, and society* (pp.182–213). New York: Guilford.

van der Straten, A., King, R., Grinstead, O., Serufilira, A., & Allen, S. (1995). Couple communication, sexual coercion and HIV risk reduction in Kigali, Rwanda. *AIDS, 9,* 935–944.

Van Oss-Marin, B., Tschann, J. M., Gomez, C. A., & Kegeles, S. M. (1993). Acculturation and gender differences in sexual attitudes and behaviors: Hispanic vs. non-Hispanic white unmarried adults. *American Journal of Public Health, 83,* 1759–1761.

Verkuyl, D. A. (1995). Practising obstetrics and gynaecology in areas with a high prevalence of HIV infection. *Lancet, 346,* 293–296.

Viney, L. L., Henry, R. M., Walker, B. M., & Crooks, L. (1992). The psychosocial impact of multiple deaths from AIDS. *Omega Journal of Death and Dying, 24* (2), 151–163.

Voeller, B. (1991). AIDS and heterosexual anal intercourse. *Archives of Sexual Behavior, 20,* 233–276.

Voeller, B., Nelson, J., & Day, C. (1994). Viral leakage risk differences in latex condoms. *AIDS Research and Human Retroviruses, 10,* 701–710.

Ward, M. C. (1993). A different disease: HIV/AIDS and health care for women in poverty. *Culture, Medicine, and Psychiatry, 17,* 413–430.

Warren, C. W., Goldberg, H. I., Oge, L., Pepion, D. Friedman, J. S., Helgerson, S., & La Mere, E. M. (1990). Assessing the reproductive behavior of on- and off-reservation American Indian females: Characteristics of two groups in Montana. *Social Biology, 37* (1–2), 69–83.

Weatherburn, P., Davies, P. M., Hickson, F. C. I., Hunt, A. J., McManus, T. J., & Coxon, A. P. M. (1993). No connection between alcohol use and unsafe sex among gay and bisexual men. *AIDS, 7,* 115–119.

Weeks, M. R., Schensul, J. J., Williams, S. S., Singer, M., & Grier, M. (1995). AIDS prevention for African-American and Latina women: Building culturally and gender-appropriate intervention. AIDS *Education and Prevention, 7,* 251–263.

Weir, S. S., Roddy, R. E., Zekeng, L., & Feldblum, P. J. (1995). Nonoxynol-9 use, genital ulcers, and HIV infection in a cohort of sex workers. *Genitourinary Medicine, 72* (2), 78–81.

Weisman, C. S., Plichta, S., Nathanson, C. A., Chase, G. A., Ensminger, M. E., & Robinson, J. C. (1991). Adolescent women's contraceptive decision-making. *Journal of Health and Social Behavior, 32,* 130–144.

Weissman, M. M., & Olfson, M. (1995, August). Depression in women: Implications for health care research. *Science, 269,* 799–801.

Wells, E. A., Hoppe, M. J., Simpson, E. E., Gillmore, M. R., Morrison, D. M., & Wilsdon, A. (1995). Misconceptions about AIDS among children who can identify the major routes of HIV transmission. *Journal of Pediatric Psychology, 20,* 671–686.

Whitbeck, L. B., Hoyt, D. R., Simons, R. L., Conger, R. D., Elder, G. H., Jr., Lorenz, F. O., & Huck, S. (1992). Intergenerational continuity of parental rejection and depressed affect. *Journal of Personality and Social Psychology, 63,* 1036–1045.

Whitbeck, L. B., Conger, R. D., & Kao, M. (1993). The influence of parental support, depressed affect, and peers on the sexual behaviors of adolescent girls. *Journal of Family Issues, 14,* 261–278.

White, G. L., Jr., Griffith, C. J., Vetrosky, D. T., & Dixon, D. (1996). Infectious vulvovaginitis: An update. *Physician Assistant, 20* (12), 41–42.

White, J. C. (1997). HIV risk assessment and prevention in lesbians and women who have sex with women: Practical information for clinicians. *Health Care for Women International, 18* (2), 127–138.

Widom, C. S. (1989). The cycle of violence. *Science, 244* (4901), 160–166.

Wilcox, B. L., Robbennolt, J. K., O'Keeffe, J. E., & Pynchon, M. E. (1996). Teen nonmarital childbearing and welfare: The gap between research and political discourse. *Journal of Social Issues, 52* (3), 71–90.

Williams, D. I., Stephenson, J. M., Hart, G. J., Copas, A., Johnson, A. M., & Williams, I. G. (1996). A case control study of HIV seroconversion in gay men, 1988–1993: What are the current risk factors? *Genitourinary Medicine, 72* (3), 193–196.

Williams, G. J. (1983). Child abuse reconsidered: The urgency of authentic prevention. *Journal of Clinical Child Psychology, 12,* 312–319.

Wilmoth, G. H., deAlteriis, M., & Bussell, D. (1992). Prevalence of psychological risks following legal abortion in the U. S.: Limits of the evidence. *Journal of Social Issues, 48* (3), 37–66.

Winter, L., & Breckenmaker, L. C. (1991). Tailoring family planning services to the special needs of adolescents. *Family Planning Perspectives, 23* (1), 24–30.

Winters, K. C., Remafedi, G., & Chan, B. Y. (1996). Assessing drug abuse among gay-bisexual young men. *Psychology of Addictive Behaviors, 10,* 228–236.

Worth, D. (1989). Sexual decision-making and AIDS: Why condom promotion among vulnerable women is likely to fail. *Studies in Family Planning, 20 ,* 297–307.

Wulfert, E., & Wan, C. K. (1993). Condom use: A self-efficacy model. *Health Psychology, 12*, 346–353.

Wyatt, G. E. (1988). The relationship between child sexual abuse and adolescent sexual functioning in Afro-American and White American women. *Annals of the New York Academy of Sciences, 528*, 11–122.

Wyatt, G. E., & Riederle, M. H. (1994). Reconceptualizing issues that affect women's sexual decision-making and sexual functioning. *Psychology of Women Quarterly, 18*, 611–625.

Wyatt, G. E., Newcomb, M. D., & Riederle, M. H. (1993). *Consensual sex and sexual abuse: Women's developmental patterns and outcomes*. Newbury Park, CA: Sage.

Yawn, B. P., & Yawn, R. A. (1993). Adolescent pregnancies in rural America: A review of the literature and strategies for primary prevention. *Family and Community Health, 16* (1), 36–45.

Zeanah, P. D., & Schwarz, J. C. (1996). Reliability and validity of the Sexual Self-Esteem Inventory for Women. *Assessment, 3* (1), 1–15.

Zuravin, S. J. (1987). Unplanned pregnancies, family planning problems, and child maltreatment. *Family Relations Journal of Applied Family and Child Studies, 36* (2), 135–139.

Zuravin, S. J., & DiBlasio, F. A. (1992). Child-neglecting adolescent mothers: How do they differ from their nonmaltreating counterparts? *Journal of Interpersonal Violence, 7*, 471–489.

Index

163